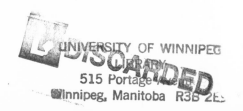

Milton's *Comus:* Family Piece

Milton's *Comus:* Family Piece

by

William B. Hunter, Jr.

The Whitston Publishing Company
Troy, New York
1983

Library of Congress Catalog Card Number 82-50824

ISBN 0-87875-257-9

Printed in the United States of America

TABLE OF CONTENTS

PREFACE

This book originated in my own feelings of inadequcy as year after year I taught *Comus* without conviction to undergraduates. I had no real problem with the rest of Milton's English poetry and could elicit responses, usually enthusiastic, from my students. But *Comus* remained an embarrassment, too obviously important to be silently ignored though I could not honestly support its ideas. Leading my classes in a skeptical attack upon them always struck me as an easy if somehow ignoble way to avoid the problem of my inability to cope with the play—one, however, to which I sometimes turned in self-defense since I had nothing affirmative to offer instead. At other times I lectured on the background of the court masque to avoid the issue.

Only after years of such apologetics did I slowly come to the understanding of Milton's play presented in this book. It has proved entirely satisfactory for both me and my students. We now read *Comus* with enthusiasm; some find it to be their favorite of Milton's work. I wish that I could correct those unenlightened discussions of earlier years, but perhaps some of those students of long ago will read this book and find in it ideas which my ignorance then prevented me from arguing with them.

The ideas in it have been a long time aborning. As over the years they reached conclusive shape I published some of them in brief notes. It is a pleasure to thank the editors of *English Language Notes* for permission to repeat here the arguments which they originally issued in quite different forms as "The Liturgical Context of *Comus*," 10 (1972), 11-15; "The Date and Occasion of *Arcades*," 11 (1973), 46-47; and "The Date of Milton's Sonnet 7," 13 (1975), 10-14. I owe the same kind of debt to *Milton Quarterly,* for "John Milton: Autobiographer," 8 (1974), 100-104, and to *Studies in English and American Literature: A Supplement to American Notes and Queries* (Troy, New York, 1978), for "Donne's 'Nocturnal' and *Isaiah* 38," pp. 85-86. There is, of course, a great deal of information in the book that follows that has never before appeared in print, but I have ignored such well-established sources or analogues as the *Odyssey* or Peele's *Old Wives Tales* if I cannot demonstrate that they have a family connection.

Finally, to two outstanding scholars I owe special thanks for help and advice. French Fogle has shared with me his extensive knowledge of Lady Alice, Countess of Derby, and her family, and his ideas about where *Comus* was staged at Ludlow. John Shawcross first suggested an elaboration of my arguments which would incorporate the several published and unpublished details into a single unit, and advised me about textual difficulties. Both helped me survive several bouts with the Dragon Error. Those rounds which I lost to it are entirely my own, which I can refer only to my own Daemon Ignorance.

Houston, Texas

ILLUSTRATIONS

of the Younger Brother. From the Tatton Park Collection, courtesy of the Courtauld Institute of Art.

6. Henry Lawes, musician, who took the part of Thyrsis. By permission of the Heather Professor of Music, Oxford University.

7. Mervin Touchet, Earl of Castlehaven and husband of Anne, Lady Alice's daughter, from the frontispiece of *The Arraignment and Conviction of Mervin Lord Audley* (1642). No paintings of him seem to have survived.

8. Ludlow Castle, the inner bailey. The recessed section is the southeast wall of the Great Hall against which *Comus* was most probably staged, also the location of the stage for modern productions. The round Norman chapel is a few yards outside the picture at the right.

Special thanks for assistance in securing the reproductions owe to John Sunderland, Witt Librarian of the Courtauld Institute of Art, and to Rosalind K. Marshall of the Scottish National Portrait Gallery.

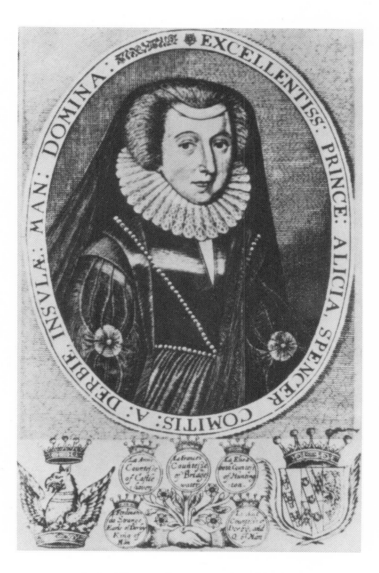

Lady Alice, Dowager Countess of Derby

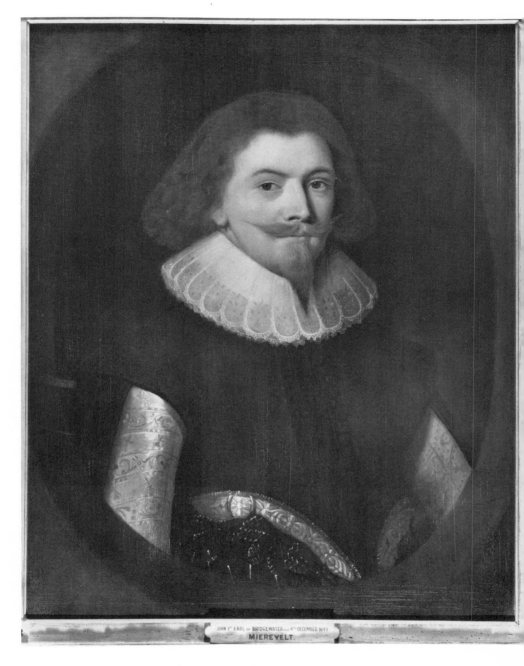

JOHN 1ST EARL OF BRIDGEWATER DIED 4TH DECEMBER 1649.
MIEREVELT.

John Egerton, First Earl of Bridgewater
Courtesy of the Courtauld Institute of Art

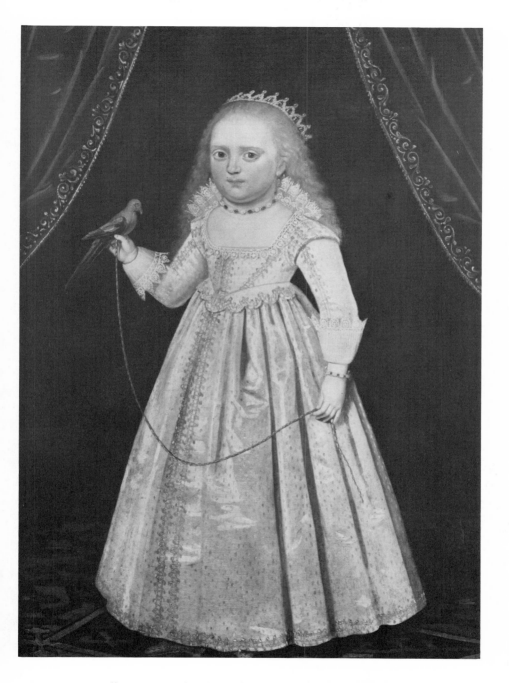

Alice Egerton, daughter of the First Earl of Bridgewater
Courtesy of the Duke of Sutherland and the Scottish National Portrait Gallery

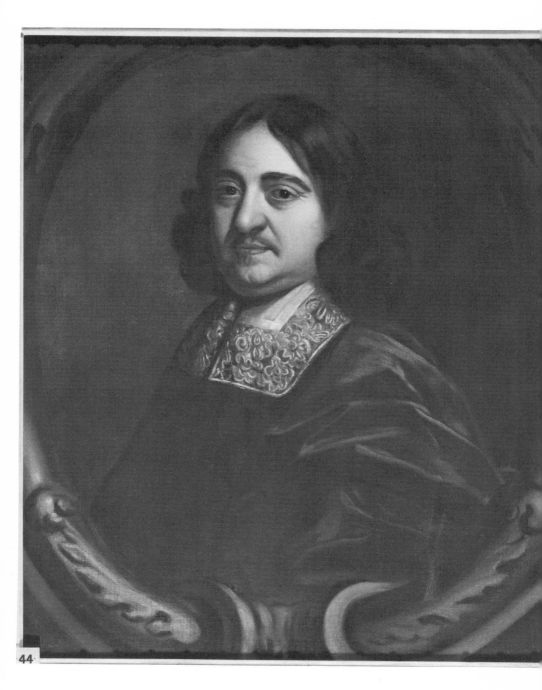

John Egerton, Second Earl of Bridgewater
Courtesy of the Courtauld Institute of Art

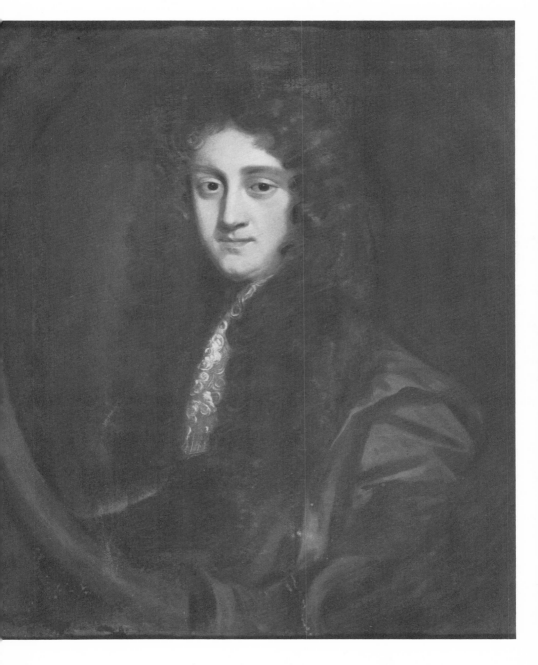

Thomas Egerton
Courtesy of the Courtauld Institute of Art

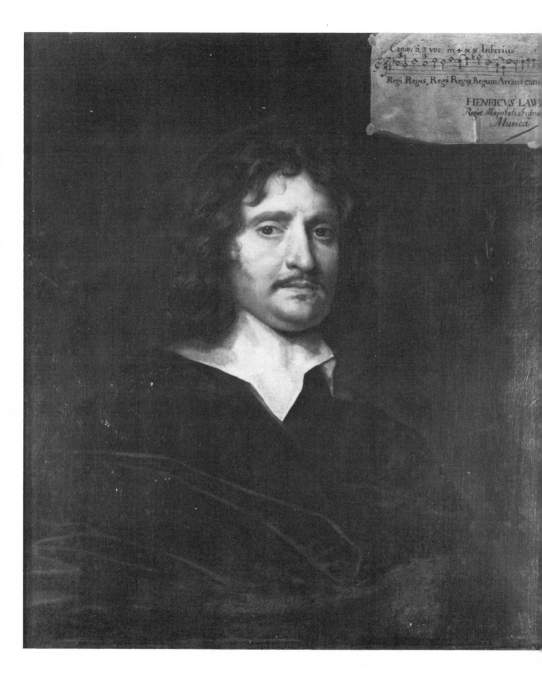

Henry Lawes
By permission of the Heather Professor of Music, Oxford University

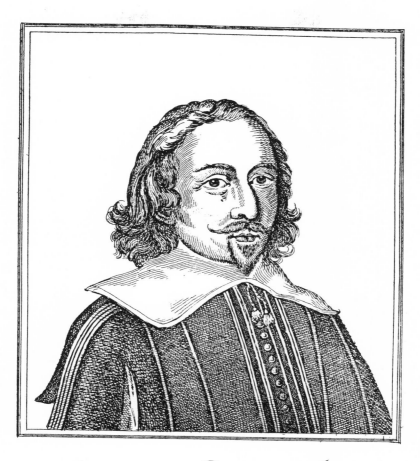

The true Portraiture of

MERVIN EARL of CASTLEHAVEN

Mervin Touchet, Earl of Castlehaven

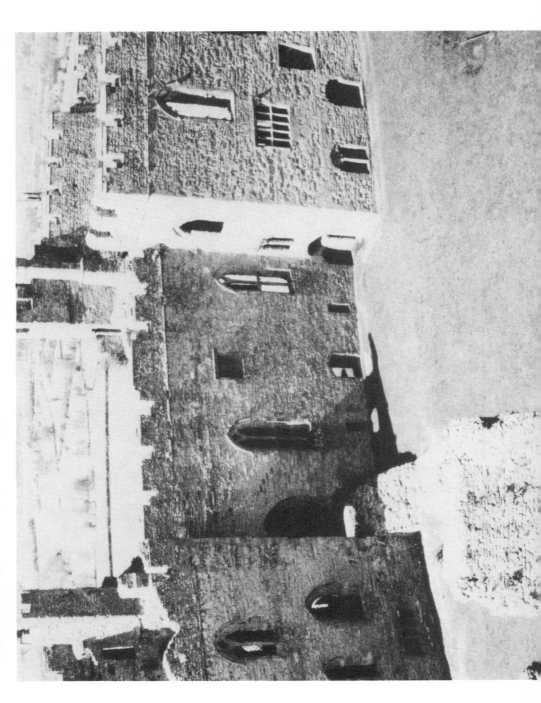

Ludlow Castle, the inner bailey

CHAPTER I

THE PROBLEM OF *COMUS*

In one respect, that of its moral contents, John Milton's masque *Comus* has not received much favorable criticism since its original production at Ludlow Castle on the evening of September 29, 1634. The reason is not far to seek: in his play Milton exalts the virtue of chastity. Wondering what will protect from danger their sister, who is lost in the "wild wood" of the opening scene, the younger brother hears from his older sibling that she has "a hidden strength: . . . 'Tis chastitie, my brother, chastitie" (433-435),[1] and he goes on to assert that no one "Will dare to soyl her virgin purity." Thus even rape itself is powerless: "no evill thing . . . Has hurtfull power ore true virginity" (446-451), a statement so at odds with the facts of life as to nonplus any audience. Even after the brothers learn from the Attendant Spirit Thyrsis that their sister has fallen under Comus's dread power, the older brother refuses to be overcome by the bad news:

> Vertue may be assail'd, but never hurt,
> Surpriz'd by unjust force, but not enthrall'd. (603-604)

The Lady had earlier reassured herself by paraphrasing St. Paul's well-known formulation of the theological virtues:

> O welcome pure-ey'd Faith, white-handed Hope . . . ,
> And thou unblemish't forme of Chastitie, (227-229)

a phrase at which many a modern critic has gagged. But later Milton re-emphasizes her confidence when, directly faced with force at the hands of Comus, the Lady reiterates her belief in

1

"the Sun-clad power of Chastity" (796). Fortunately, our credulity is not put to test by the actuality: her brothers rush in and rescue her.

For an age like our own which all too often must confront the bitter and psychologically destructive fact of rape, this central message of *Comus* has only an empty ring. It is at best well-intended moralizing, at worst the public confession of its author's own sexual problems. Nor is our generation alone. Alvin Thaler has pointed out that the play was performed well over two hundred times in the eighteenth century with various modifications which sometimes, like John Dalton's operatic form, made "vice as seductive, and virtue as stupid, as possible."[2] Unwilling to accept its central moral message in view of the realities of life, readers usually turn to *Comus* for the beauty of its poetry, which is certainly there, just as many read the Bible for the same reason. But the Bible exists first of all for its contents: Koheleth, for example, had something important that he wanted to say, and the fact that he said it beautifully in Ecclesiastes is in one sense an accident. Medium and message certainly cannot be separated, but a medium without an acceptable message or with one so apparently flawed as that of *Comus* appears to be becomes in time for its reader not much more than white noise. But this seems to be the way that the play is usually read today, primarily for the very real beauty of its lines or because of the reputation which its author well deserves for his other writings—not for its moral contents, which are downright embarrassing to discuss seriously.

When confronted by this aesthetic problem which *Comus* so expressly poses, twentieth century critics have tended to interpret it as they have interpreted much of the rest of Milton's poetry, as autobiographical statements: the play's thesis of the power of chastity and virginity, that is, is a public affirmation of its author's own private beliefs. One cannot gainsay the fundamental importance of such an approach to his writing, for like many other Christians of that day he seems to have examined every event in his life to find in it a manifestation of God's grace to him,[3] and in this sense he put himself frequently into both his prose and his verse. Anti-Miltonists see such self-interest as mere egotism, but this does not do him justice. He certainly found himself an interesting subject, and to ignore this

2

fact is to deprive oneself of much of the impact of, say, *Lycidas* and the Sonnets, although the extent of autobiography in *Samson Agonistes* is still being argued.

Even more important in the case of *Comus* is the clear evidence provided in some of his other works upon which critics have based their arguments for an autobiographical reading of the sexual issues underlying the play. Saurat, Hanford, and Tillyard, for instance, all join to emphasize the important self-confession which Milton wrote into his *Apology against a Pamphlet* in 1642 and which they retrospectively apply to *Comus.*[4] Arguing from Revelation 14. 1-5, whose author places those "which were not defiled with women"—male virgins—singing before the Throne of God, and from several passages in 1 Corinthians, Milton outlines his own personal development to his opponents:

> having had the doctrine of holy Scripture unfolding those chaste and high mysteries with timeliest care infus'd, that *the body is for the Lord and the Lord for the body,* thus also I argu'd to my selfe; that if unchastity in a woman whom Saint *Paul* termes the glory of man, be such a scandall and dishonour, then certainly in a man who is both the image of glory of God, it must, though commonly not so thought, be much more deflouring and dishonourable. In that he sins both against his owne body which is the perfecter sex, and his own glory which is in the woman, and that which is worst, against the image and glory of God which is in himselfe.[5]

Even though he published these sentences some eight years after he wrote *Comus* and may have changed his moral standards in that time, there is no good reason to doubt that Milton had always put a high value on chastity. With Strabo he seems from early years to have thought that the good poet must first be a good man. In a famous statement, he concluded,

> I was confirm'd in this opinion, that he who would not be frustrate of his hope to write well hereafter in laudable things, ought him selfe to bee a true Poem, that is, a composition, and patterne of the best and honourablest things; not presuming to sing high praises of heroick men, or famous Cities, unlesse he have in himselfe the experience and the practice of all that which is praise-worthy.[6]

As Tillyard observed, "such ideas [of chastity] had been exercising his mind [at the time of the composition of *Comus*], and were to exercise it for some years to come."[7] With the kind of evidence which has been cited lesser critics find the author's own

3

concerns at the heart of the play, and very nearly every one reads it to some degree as a personal document or confession. Such an approach reaches its extreme statement in Malcolm Ross's exclamation, "Faith, Hope, and *Chastity*. And the greatest of these is chastity! The substitution of chastity for charity is the reduction of the highest supernatural grace to a secondary practical virtue."[8] As the editor of the Variorum rightly protests, such an overreading seems "to have exchanged the text of *Comus for Pamela*."[9]

But a fact which has not hitherto been accorded sufficient recognition is that Milton wrote the play on commission directly or ultimately from John Egerton, the Earl of Bridgewater, as part of the celebration of his inauguration as Lord President of Wales. This being the case, nothing could be further from the truth than Leishman's statement that in its composition Milton was "given a completely free hand,"[10] for the commissioning of masques did not work that way. Rather, Parker is correct in observing that "nothing else that [Milton] ever wrote was so thoroughly influenced by the wishes of others and by external circumstances. It was limited from the outset by certain practical considerations utterly beyond his control."[11] Indeed, the writer of a masque had to do exactly as he was told, for any significant deviations that were not welcome would, of course, have been recognized and changed or deleted by the participants in the rehearsals. Here, for instance, is Ben Jonson's description of how he composed his *Masque of Beauty* in 1608. Plans for the occasion originated with Queen Anne, he writes, who directed that he should continue and extend the ideas of his previous *Masque of Blackness,* adding four participants to the group of masquers disguised as Negroes but keeping to the same general subject of showing them as they seek out a place (Egnland) where they may find Beauty. Accordingly, Jonson "apted" his invention to achieve the effects which the Queen had commanded.[12] Indeed, for him to have done otherwise would have been to court disaster. As a matter of fact, Henry Lawes, who played the part of Thyrsis in *Comus* and undoubtedly provided the liaison between the Egerton family and Milton, himself wrote in his letter dedicating the 1637 edition of the play to John Viscount Brackley, "Son and Heir apparent to the Earl of *Bridgewater, &c.*" that the work "receiv'd its first occasion of Birth from your Self, and others of your Noble Family," with the implication that the family had

4

originally directed what the subject was to be (and it must have included a statement that three of their children would be active participants; Lawes goes on to praise John for his performance as the Elder Brother). This is not to say that the family dictated the plot itself or that it specified any or all of its details, the music which Lawes was to compose for it, or how the whole was to be produced. But it does mean that whoever commissioned the entertainment for the evening of September 29, either the Earl or his agent, directed what the general subject would be. A surprising if obvious fact is that Milton was told not to center his play upon the occasion, Bridgewater's installation as Lord President of Wales or upon the topic of Wales itself: only the Prologue and restoration of the children to their parents mentions the former, and only Sabrina as the River Severn even obliquely the latter. Instead, the Earl evidently directed that the topic would be the family itself as three of its younger members would participate in the performance and that instead of glorification of some aspect of the occasion the subject would be the vindication of family virtue as their youngest daughter confronted temptation and assault. Traditional though the subject of chastity was in the literature of the period, it is something of an unexpected center of this particular public ceremony. But the last thing that Bridgewater and his guests would find acceptable on such a festive occasion would be the revelations of the sexual hang-ups of their author, as some critics would have one believe.

At the same time, one must recognize that Milton found the directive to be entirely congenial with those judgments which he would express later in his *Apology;* indeed, he may have responded too enthusiastically for the family tastes. The *Comus* text survives in three early and distinctive forms: The Trinity Manuscript, so called because it is in the Trinity College Library at Cambridge; the Bridgewater Manuscript, named for the family; and the first edition of the work, which Lawes printed in 1637. For various reasons too complex to enter into here, the Bridgewater text seems closer to the 1634 performance than do either of the others; but it cuts three major sections of the play which appear in the others—lines 209-239 (the Lady's soliloquy on chastity) and 751-769 (Comus's argument against virginity), both of which are in the Trinity Manuscript and 1637, and 793-820 (the Lady's most explicit defense of chastity), which first appears in 1637.

5

Now it happens that these passages deal more expressly and forcefully with the subject of chastity than does any of the rest of the play. Were they written before the performance, as some think, and deleted from it because of family tastes, or were they added by Milton some time after the performance as others argue?[13] As will appear below, it seems probably that the first example is a true excision of material written before the performance and deleted from it at least as much because of exegencies of stage presentation as because of its moral contents. There is no certainty about whether the second was cut before the performance to accord with family wishes or added by Milton after it. As for the third, since it is absent from both manuscripts and first appears in the 1637 edition, it may be Milton's own later addition. In any case they all three may testify as much to the author's as to the family's high evaluation of chastity. This emphasis, however, must not be permitted to obscure the subject of family virtue which dominates all of the play and which must have been the substance of the Earl's original directive.

It is not clear whether the family or the poet decided on the contents of the parts assigned to each of the children, but the results as they stand must have pleased everyone. The Lady—Alice, the youngest daughter—would defend her own virtue against the arguments of Comus by demonstrating how specious they were, her own morality being the central issue. The Younger Brother, Thomas, doubts the efficacy of chastity in the real world ("Doubting Thomas"?). Finally, rather than the mature Thyrsis the Older Brother John, then aged 11, carries the full responsibility for stating the case of the generalized efficacy of morality. For instance,

> against the threats
> Of malice or sorcerie, or that power
> Which erring men call Chance, this I hold firme,
> Vertue may be assailed'd, but never hurt,
> Surpriz'd by unjust force, but not enthrall'd,
> Yea even that which mischiefe meant most harme,
> Shall in the happie triall prove most glorie.
> But evill on it selfe shall backe recoyle
> And mixe no more with goodnesse, when at last
> Gather'd like scum, and setl'd to it selfe
> It shall bee in eternall restlesse change
> Selfe, fed, and selfe consum'd.   600-611

6

That evening in late September as it heard these lines, the audience would constantly be aware of the fact that their spokesman was the oldest son and heir of the family—the future Earl of Bridgewater—representing his father and his entire family.

A simple if unusual example will show just how clearly Milton kept the Bridgewater family in mind as he "apted his invention" and wrote his dialogue. In those days both forms of the second person singular pronoun were in active use: thou/thine/thee to be addressed to those of lower social status, you/yours, for equals or superiors. The social ranks hold even within Milton's masque for the people taking its acting roles. Thus despite his evident chronological seniority and general expansiveness, Comus in or out of "disguise" unfailingly addresses the Lady with the formal pronoun *you*, as a servant should. She in turn always addresses him as *thou*. Thyrsis (Lawes, who taught the children music) likewise addresses her as *you* in recognition of his social role with a young lady now reaching adulthood. Only Sabrina, a goddess, can address her as *thou* when she removes the spell holding the Lady in her chair, in a speech really more incantation than direct address. On the other hand, Thyrsis speaks to the boys and they to him as *thou* (after his identity becomes clear to them; until then they employ the formal *you*, which is proper for a stranger), the familiar pronoun suggesting something of their youth as the formal one recognizes the maturity of their sister Alice. He, of course, always uses the plural *you* or *ye* when speaking to the boys jointly; they always employ the polite *you* to one another, as young gentlemen should. Milton knew the code of courtly diction and followed it.

In conclusion, one may be certain that as he responded to the family directive for the masque Milton's efforts were entirely successful. Lawes said as much as he continued the letter to young John cited above: the poem is "so lovely, and so much desired, that the often Copying of it hath tir'd my Pen." But why should the Egerton family have defined so unusual a subject for the inaugural entertainment, and how did Milton go about obliging them? To discover the answers to such questions, it is necessary first to see how he had earlier that year created a much simpler entertainment, that for the Dowager Countess of Derby, mother-in-law and step-mother to the Earl of Bridgewater. He named it *Arcades.*

7

NOTES

[1] Unless otherwise indicated all quotations from Milton's text refer to the reconstructed, composite one printed below in Chapter VI.

[2] "Milton in the Theatre," *SP*, 17 (1920), 291.

[3] See my "John Milton: Autobiographer," *MQ*, 8 (1974), 1001-104.

[4] Denis Saurat, *Milton: Man and Thinker* (New York, 1925), p. 9; James Holly Hanford, "The Youth of Milton," *Studies in Shakespeare, Milton, and Donne by Members of the English Department of the University of Michigan* (New York, 1925), p. 143; E. M. W. Tillyard, *Milton* (London, 1946), Appendix C.

[5] Edited by Frederick L. Taft in *Complete Prose Works of John Milton*, 1 (1953), 892.

[6] *Complete Prose Works*, p. 890.

[7] Tillyard, p. 381.

[8] *Poetry and Dogma* (New Brunswick, New Jersey, 1954), p. 196.

[9] *A Variorum Commentary on the Poems of John Milton*, 2 (New York, 1972), 808.

[10] J. B. Leishman, *Milton's Minor Poems* (Pittsburgh, 1969), p. 165. As for the "sage and serious doctrine of virginity," Milton seems to him to be speaking "*in propria persona*," p. 199.

[11] William R. Parker, *Milton: A Biography* (Oxford, 1968), I, 128. Rosemary Mundhenk emphasizes this point of view and anticipates in part

the thesis of the present study in her "Dark Scandal and the Sun-Clad Power of Chastity: The Historical Milieu of Milton's *Comus*," *SEL*, 15 (1975), 141-153.

[12]See my edition of the masque in *The Complete Poetry of Ben Jonson* (New York: 1963), p. 414.

[13]S. E. Sprott supports a pre-performance date for the composition of all three passages in *John Milton, A Maske: The Earlier Versions* (Toronto, 1973), p. 5, a book which conveniently prints all three versions in parallel format. John Shawcross has argued that they are additions made later: "Certain Relationships of the Manuscripts of *Comus*," *PBSA* 54 (1960), 38, 293-294; "Speculations on the Dating of the Trinity MS of Milton's Poems," *MLN*, 75 (1960), 11-17.

CHAPTER II

THE CREATION OF *ARCADES*

No one knows for sure how the young Milton came to the attention of the family of the Dowager Countess of Derby. He certainly was not widely known as a writer, having actually published only sixteen lines of poetry, and that anonymously: "On Shakespeare," prefixed to the second folio of Shakespeare's works in 1632. The record makes it abundantly clear that its future opponent was at this time planning a career as a member of the Establishment. As a Cambridge undergraduate he had praised such of its public leaders as the late Bishops of Ely and Winchester. He had written a whole series of epigrams in Latin and one long poem, "In Quintum Novembris," to commemorate the uncovering of the Gunpowder Plot and thus indirectly to exalt the King. More recently, he had written a fine epitaph on the Marchioness of Winchester, a wealthy heiress, possibly on invitation for a memorial volume to her which never appeared. On or near his twenty-third birthday in 1631 he wrote a sonnet in which he evaluated his situation.

Having almost completed his master's degree, an effort which in his case would normally lead to his being ordained into the church (but surely as a university fellow, not as a pulpit priest), Milton found his way blocked to ecclesiastical preferment. In the ordinary course of events he would have been ordained deacon shortly after his twenty-third birthday and priest a year later.[1] But to be ordained, the candidate had to have in view, according to the then controlling Church Canons of 1604, "some certain place where he might use his function." Milton was offered none, and so he was never ordained. In the sonnet he professes himself disappointed, lacking, he observes with some irony, that "inward ripeness" which "som more timely-happy spirits indu'th," as they move along to their normal ordination. He goes on to conclude he must learn to live with the fact as an expression of God's will:

> All is, if I have grace to use it so,
> As ever in my great task-maisters eye.

The sonnet does not, however, evince any bitterness toward the established church nor does a letter which he wrote some time later to a yet-unidentified friend who had questioned him about his plans for a career.[2] Indeed, only when he had finally cut all his ties with the Establishment, some ten years later, did he conclude bitterly that he had been "Church-outed by the Prelats" who had not given him that preferment which he now in retrospect felt that he had deserved.[3] But everything known about Milton in 1634 shows that he still considered himself attached to the ruling group in which King Charles was head of both the Church and the body politic, and the Derbys and Bridgewaters were major luminaries. In this respect, his career to this point somewhat parallels that of George Herbert, who before and after he was ordained seems to have sought political preferment and only later, accepting the fact that he would not be successful at court, devoted himself instead to the appointment at Bemerton.

Although we do not know how Milton happened to be associated with such prominent people as the Egertons, he may have been brought to their attention through his poem commemorating the Marchioness of Winchester; for her father, Thomas Viscount Savage, and the Bridgewaters owned property in the same county, Cheshire. Another guess is that it came about through friendship with the musician Henry Lawes, who taught the Bridgewater children music and who wrote the music for *Comus* and took the part of its Attendant Spirit Thyrsis. If the latter, the best guess as to how Milton met Lawes is that Lawes and Milton's father had become friends through their mutual commitment to music, which would have brought them together in the musical society of London.[4] But we really do not know for certain how poet and musician met, though it is perfectly clear that they became friends and remained so even through the strains of the Civil War when they supported opposite sides.

It is also a guess, but now a very likely one, that Lawes took the part of the Genius of the Wood in *Arcades*. The part is quite similar to the one of the Attendant Spirit which he certainly took in *Comus*, as the conclusion of his letter to the young John Viscount Brackley already cited testifies, and it involves shepherding several young participants, some of them his music students, through the simple actions of the entertainment as he was to do later in the much more complex *Comus*. In both he presents them to the persons being acclaimed, and in both he sings.

The ceremony of which *Arcades* was a part was planned to honor the Dowager Countess of Derby at her country estate, Harefield. As would later be the case in *Comus*, the person or persons planning the celebration undoubtedly gave Milton directions as to what the general subject and tone should be. From what he wrote one can be sure that the directive was a simple one: loving recognition of the grand old lady by her family.

Indeed, Alice, the Countess, was a grand old lady. Born on Holy Thursday, 1559, to Sir John Spencer of Althorpe, ancestor of today's Lady Diana Spencer, she had married Ferdinando Stanley, Lord Strange and later Earl of Derby, in 1579. He became noted as a friend of writers and was himself a poet. Edmund Spenser claimed to be a relative of Alice and dedicated his *Teares of the Muses* to her; she is also the "Amaryllis" of his *Colin Clouts Come Home Again* and its "Amyntas" is Ferdinando. He in turn was a friend of the Earl of Essex, one of Shakespeare's benefactors, and patron of an acting company, Lord Strange's Men, who certainly staged at least *Titus Andronicus* and very probably other early plays of Shakespeare.

Besides being a relative of the Tudors, descended through his mother from a sister of Henry VII, Ferdinando was also a king of sorts in his own right: he was "King" of the Isle of Man. The title goes back to the days of Henry IV. When Henry returned from exile to overthrow Richard II the island was ruled by the Earl of Wiltshire, whom Henry promptly had executed without trial, as readers of Shakespeare's play will remember. In his place he assigned Henry Percy (Hotspur), but when he defected, Henry, according to William Camden's history,

> sent Sir *John Stanley,* and *William Stanley* to seize the isle and
> castle of Man, the inheritance whereof hee granted afterward to
> Sir *John Stanley,* and his heirs, by Letters Patent with the Pat-
> ronage of the Bishopricke &c.   And so his heirs and successours.
> Who[ever] were honoured [with] the title of Earles of Derby,
> were commonly called *Kings of Man.*[5]

In the last decade of the sixteenth century the fifth Earl was
Ferdinando Stanley, King of Man and Alice's husband. It may be
significant to observe that she retained the title of Countess of
Derby after his death in 1594 and even after her remarriage in
1600.

To continue the record of her literary associations, she was
praised by Thomas Nashe; John Marston wrote a masque in her
honor, and French Fogle has informed me that he has identified
her as having danced in at least one of Jonson's masques, *Beauty*
(1608) and almost certainly in its predecessor, *Blackness* (1605).
Jonson named a "Co. of Derbye" as third in the list of twelve
court ladies who participated in the former.   Previously this
Countess has been identified with Elizabeth, wife of Alice's
brother-in-law William, who succeeded to the title on the death
of Ferdinando.   But recently John Orrell has discovered a rare
publication by an eye-witness to the performance of *Beauty,* an
Italian poem by Antimo Galli, who expressly praises an "Alicia
Darbi" as one of the masquers.[6]   In the forthcoming publication
of his Clark Seminar paper Fogle identifies "Alicia" as the
Countess Dowager, concluding that "this finally pins down the
identity of the Countess of Derby among the ladies who participated," and he thinks that she is the same Countess of Derby
in *Blackness* because "Jonson himself says the ladies were the
same in the two masques."

Besides this relationship, Jonson addressed several poems
to Alice's second husband, Sir Thomas Egerton, later to be Lord
Chancellor Ellesmere.   Donne was secretary for a time to Sir
Thomas and wrote a number of poems to his step-daughter,
Alice's youngest child Elizabeth, who had married Henry Hast-
ings, Earl of Huntingdon.   John Davies of Hereford dedicated
his *Holy Roode* to her in 1609 as did Thomas Gainsforde his

14

Historie of Trebizonde in 1616.[7]   Who else can claim direct relationships with Spenser, Shakespeare, Jonson, Donne, and
Milton? Indeed in the 1630's Alice was a grand old lady, and it
seems only fitting that the young Milton should be the last
writer to honor her with a poem.[8]

In *Arcades* he responds to the occasion with conventional
praise expressed especially in three magnificent songs. Some of
his emphasis, however, turns slightly away from the Countess to
praise her descendents, her daughters and grandchildren who
participated in the celebration. Milton's concern was to under-
score how they evince "bright honor." The reason for the emphasis upon the nobility of the children hardly requires comment as indirect praise of their distinguished ancestor, though
full understanding of the importance of asserting the purity of
the family name in them must await a later chapter. A more
oblique reference is his praise of Alice as "the wise *Latona*"
(19), for Latona was, of course, mother of Diana, goddess of
chastity. A final point that may be worthy of mention is the fact
that, as William Camden observes, the name *Alice* derives from
Germanic *Adeliz,* meaning *noble.*[9] Milton may intend recognition of the meaning of her name when the Genius invites "ye
. . . all that are of noble stemm" (82) to approach her "state."

Because the festivities took place at her rural seat, Harefield, Milton conventionally associated it with rural Arcadia,
famous in classical myth for its pastoral contentment. In ad-
dressing Alice twice as "rural Queen" he may have had in mind
her former title associated with the Isle of Man; she herself at
least might be expected to recognize the reference. As several
critics have observed, Milton quite possibly had visited the
estate. *Arcades* is set there out of doors, where the children,
guided by the "genius of the Wood," approach the "state"
where Alice is seated. Thus in his second song the Genius leads
the children over the greensward up the avenue to her:

> O're the smooth enameld green
> Where no print of step hath been,
> > Follow me as I sing,
> > And touch the warbled string
> Under the shady roof
> Of branching Elm Star-proof,

> Follow me,
>   I will bring you where she sits
>   Clad in splendor as befits
>   Her deity.

Milton seems to have known that they would come up an avenue of elms known as the "Queen's Walk," named from the reception of Queen Elizabeth on it in a similar entertainment in 1602,[10] and he seems to have known that the house was located on a hill, for the Genius says that in caring for it

>   I fetch my round
>   Over the mount, and all this hallow'd ground.   (54-55)

One of Milton's most interesting personal applications occurs in the second stanza of the first song:

> *Fame* that her high worth to raise
> Seem'd erst so lavish and profuse,
> We may justly now accuse
> Of detraction from her praise,
>   Less then half we find exprest,
>   *Envy* bid conceal the rest.

As John M. Wallace has pointed out,[11] Milton here is adapting to his own purposes the description of the visit of the Queen of Sheba to King Solomon in 1 Kings 10.6-7:

> And she said to the king, It was a true report that I heard in mine own land of thy acts and of thy wisdom. Howbeit I believed not the words, until I came, and mine eyes had seen it; and, behold, the half was not told me: thy wisdom and prosperity exceedeth the fame which I heard.

There are other reflections of this chapter as well: the description of Solomon's throne in verses 18 to 20 suggests the "shining throne" of line 16 in which Alice was seated and her "glittering state" of line 81. And, of course, her comparison with the "wise *Latona*" (19) already mentioned in another context, suggests one of Solomons' most famous attributes.

Granted that these parallels become obvious when printed

side by side in this way, they seem otherwise obscure. The implicit identification of Solomon's being greeted by an adulatory Queen of Sheba in 1 Kings 10 with Alice's being greeted by her adoring relations in the performance itself would seem to have been quite impossible for anyone to recognize except a highly knowledgeable and perceptive student of the Bible. But there is one means by which Milton would have known in advance that the parallel would be brought to the attention of the audience so that they would certainly make the association.

Then as now communicants of the Church of England participated in the daily religious services of Morning Prayer and Evening Prayer. A section of each has always required the reading of passages from the Old Testament and from the New Testament specified for each day in the year, during which the whole Bible would be pretty well covered. These "lessons" for each day (and for each special holy day) were printed in a Calendar prefixed to the Prayer Book. (It should be mentioned that in 1662 the daily readings were somewhat altered so that a modern Calendar cannot be depended on for the readings of the 1630's.) It is a rather eerie fact that today one can determine for any given day in Milton's time exactly what biblical passages a communicant would hear during these services. Generally speaking, the readings for Evening Prayer of the night before seem to be most significant for any given date. Thus when John Donne wrote in his "A nocturnall upon *S. Lucies day*" (December 13 by his calendar) that "my Sunne" will not "renew"—that is, return—most readers understand him to be referring to his dead wife or to his hopes in life, and so he may indeed. At the same time one must remember that as an ordained priest he participated actively in worship services. A few hours earlier on the night of December 12 he would have read in the service Isaiah 38, prescribed as the first lesson for Evening Prayer on that day. It narrates how good King Hezekiah faced death from an illness. Isaiah at his side, however, tells him that his prayers have been answered and that he will live fifteen years longer. Because the King is skeptical the prophet gives him a "sign": the shadow of the sun miraculously moves backwards ten degrees: Hezekiah's sun "returns." Donne, in utter despair, has no hope of such a promise.[1][2]

The application of the Calendar to explain biblical references in certain poems in English literature of this period can thus produce interesting insights as their authors participated in the daily readings. Mother Christopher Pecheux has demonstrated their applicability to the "Ode on the Morning of Christ's Nativity."[13] They lie so obviously back of the poems for January 1 ("The Circumcision") and Good Friday ("The Passion") as to require very little comment. In the second stanza of the former poem, for instance, Milton employs (line 21) the idea of a convenant which God established with mankind at the institution of the rite of circumcision according to Genesis 17. This is the assigned first lesson for the morning service on January 1—not that Milton himself would have required such a reminder, but he would have expected his readers to recognize the relationship between his poem and the reading for the day.

It even is possible to apply the principle to Milton's understanding of the direction his own life was to take. He was born on December 9, 1608. The New Testament lesson for the night before was the first chapter of the Epistle of James. In this important passage temptation is a central issue—"Blessed is the man that endureth temptation" (vs. 12)—the subject of all four of Milton's major poems. It is the biblical source (vs. 15) of the allegory of Sin and Death in *Paradise Lost.* And it is the main biblical statement of how important it is that a Christian express his faith in action: "Be ye doers of the word, and not hearers only" (vs. 22), going on the emphasize as Milton himself would later "the perfect law of liberty," though one must "keep himself unspotted from the world." Here is an almost perfect characterization of Milton's own life as it developed, of his concern for his own chastity, and of his developing Arminianism which in time led to his role as a political and religious activist.[14] We know that he was interested in his birthdays. He wrote a poem about one of them, the sonnet already discussed, which seems ultimately to be his response at that time to the demands of the first chapter of the Epistle of James.

Thus if the household at Harefield was made up of God-fearing people (and only one, its senior member, had to be so to assure attendance at Evening Prayer), it seems safe to assume that they would all have participated in the service on the night before the celebrations in honor of Alice to which *Arcades* would contribute. All that Milton needed to know in advance was the date if he wished to allude in his planned "Entertainment" to a biblical passage which he would know that everyone would recognize. As has been seen, he referred in the second stanza of the first song to 1 Kings 10. On what date did the Calendar direct that it be read? It is assigned to Evening Prayer on May 2, a date that does not seem to be intrinsically significant until one realizes that the birthday of Alice, the person being honored, was Holy Thursday. This was not the Maundy Thursday of Holy week, but Ascension Day, forty days after Easter. In 1569, her birth year, this fell on May 4.

Now the association between May 2, with its reading from 1 Kings 10, and May 4, the birthday, seems too close to be coincidental. If the birthday were the third, there would be no problem, of course, but the reading suggests that for some reason or other the celebration was moved up one day to the eve rather than the birthday itself. The most obvious and most likely is that May 4 fell on a Sunday and the birthday celebration was accordingly transferred to Saturday. But why? If the Egerton family had had Puritan leanings the change could be explained (indeed, if they had been strong Puritans there would have been no entertainment), but they were not. In his *Book of Sport* (1633), King Charles had "prohibited all unlawful games to be used upon Sundays onely, as Beare and Bull baitings, Interludes, and . . . Bowling" (p. 12), but it is difficult to classify *Arcades* with such rowdy pastimes. More likely, as Milton describes it as only "part of an entertainment presented to the Countess Dowager," the family did not view the entire celebration as appropriate for Sunday. A piece of evidence from a generation earlier is suggestive too. In June 1603 Jonson had written an "Entertainment" for the welcome of the new Queen Anne and her son Prince Henry at Althorpe, the family seat of Alice's parents, the Spencers. That celebration began on Saturday the 25th and reached a climax when "a brace of choice Deere [were] put out, and as fortunately kill'd, as they were meant to be." But then, Jonson reports, "the next day being Sunday, [the Queen] rested," and the conclusion of this entertainment put off until "Monday . . . after dinner."[15] Similar scruples may have still prevailed in the 1630's, or the family had other plans. In any case, they moved the birthday celebration up a day to Saturday.

19

But if Milton were indeed writing under a directive for May 3 and consequently paraphrased the Calendar reading for the evening of May 2 which he would expect everyone to recognize the next day, when in the 1630's did May 4 fall on a Sunday? Every year from 1630 to 1634 has been suggested for a performance of *Arcades,* though there is no solid proof for any (since it preceded *Comus* it must antedate September 29, 1634). During this period Sunday fell on May 4 only in 1634. Easter had come on April 6, the same as it would in 1980, and May 4 was the Sunday four weeks later.[16] *Arcades* accordingly was most probably performed on Saturday, May 3, 1634, something over four months before *Comus* was produced, to celebrate Alice's seventy-fifth birthday. That the entertainment was entirely successful there is positive proof in that its author was commissioned to write a much more elaborate work for a much more important ceremony the following September, the work that he was to entitle merely *A Maske.* It must accordingly have been written rapidly, being completed during the summer of 1634. No wonder its two surviving manuscripts and two printed texts show its author making some later revisions.

What of the text of the second reading, taken from the New Testament, on that evening of May 2? The calendar directs that it be the first chapter of Romans. In *Arcades* Milton makes no mention of it at all. In it are these well-known verses:

> God has given the unrighteous unto vile affections: for even their women did change the natural use into that which is against nature: and likewise also the men, leaving the natural use of the woman, burned in their lust one toward another; men with men working that which is unseemly, and receiving in themselves that recompense of their error which was meet.

Not only does Milton avoid any reference to them, but one can be quite certain that the priest did not read these verses during the service, for they had proved bitterly appropriate in the history of the family. To discover why it now is necessary to turn from the clear serenity of Arcadia to the dark family chapter of rape and sodomy which lie back of the exaltation of chastity in *Comus.*

NOTES

[1] See my argument in "The Date of Milton's Sonnet 7," *ELN*, 13 (1975), 12-14.

[2] Milton composed it and then revised it sometime after completing *Arcades*—as will appear below almost three years after writing the sonnet, although most scholars have thought that the letter came much sooner after the poem, which he mentions as having been done "some while since." Many, too, have accepted Parker's erroneous dating of the sonnet in 1632 rather than in 1631 when he actually celebrated his twenty-third birthday and had to confront his failure to be ordained as his classmates were. For a list of the latter see my essay cited above. For texts of both versions of the letter see the Scolar Press facsimile, *John Milton: Poems, Reproduced in Facsimile from the Manuscript in Trinity College, Cambridge* (Menston, 1970). Because *Arcades* is the first entry in the manuscript, the date of its composition is basic for determining an earliest date for materials in that manuscript.

[3] *Reason of Church Government*, edited by Ralph A. Haug, *Complete Prose Works*, I, 823.

[4] The best study is that by Willa M. Evans, *Henry Lawes: Musician and Friend of Poets* (New York, 1941).

[5] *Britain*, trans. Philemon Holland (London, 1610), "British Ilands," p. 412. Queen Elizabeth II even today is titled "King of Man."

[6] "Antimo Galli's Description of *The Masque of Beauty*," *HLQ*, (1979), 13-23. See *Rime Di Antimo Galli All' Illvstrissima Signiora Ilizabetta Talbot-Grey* (London, 1609), p. 20 (misnumbered 19).

[7] Several of these works, including this one, are listed in the inven-

tory of the library of her daughter, Lady Frances, in 1627. See Alix Egerton's edition of *Comus* (1910).

[8] All of Milton's biographers, of course, devote some space to her. See for what is still one of the best David Masson, *The Life of John Milton* I (1881), 587 ff.

[9] *Remaines Concerning Britaine* (London, 1637), p. 93, with reference to its masculine equivalent, *Ethelbert,* p. 68.

[10] Masson, I, 595.

[11] "Milton's *Arcades,*" in *Milton: Modern Essays in Criticism,* ed. Arthur E. Barker (New York, 1965), pp. 77 ff.

[12] See my note in *Studies in English and American Literature: A Supplement to American Notes and Queries,* ed. John L. Cutler and Lawrence S. Thompson (Troy, New York, 1978), pp. 85-86.

[13] "The Image of the Sun in Milton's 'Nativity Ode'," *HLQ,* 38 (1975), 315-333.

[14] See my "John Milton: Autobiographer," cited above.

[15] *Ben Jonson,* ed. C. H. Herford and Percy Simpson, 7 (Oxford, 1941), 128. Milton, incidentally, seems to have studied this entertainment, for as several critics have observed he applies the greeting to Anne,

> This is shee
>
> This is shee

to Alice in his opening song, perhaps expecting her to recognize the phase from an occasion in which she quite possibly had participated.

[16] Information about dates may be most conveniently derived from Tables I and III of Appendix IV in Paul Harvey, *The Oxford Companion to English Literature,* 3rd edition (Oxford, 1946). See also my note, "The Date and Occasion of *Arcades,*" *ELN,* 11 (1973), 46-47. As I report there, the account books of the manager of the Harefield estate survive in the Huntington Library. They begin just one week too late to verify the date argued here, a tantalizing disappointment.

CHAPTER III

THE FAMILY BACKGROUND OF *COMUS*

As has already been mentioned, Alice, the Countess of Derby, lost her husband Ferdinando in 1594. At the age of thirty-five he died rather suddenly. According to the annalist John Stow, on the night of April 4 he dreamed that Lady Alice was dangerously ill. The next day he himself was struck down; Stow thought that a witch did him in. The historian had an eye for details: having vomited fifty-two times and having passed no urine after April 12 despite heroic efforts on the part of his physicians, Ferdinando died on April 16.[1] Dugdale and others suspected poison, for as a relative of the Tudors some Jesuits may have besought him to overthrow Elizabeth and killed him for their own safety when he refused.[2] He left his widow Alice with three daughters: Anne, the oldest, Frances, and Elizabeth.

In 1600 the widow married a widower, the Lord Keeper, Sir Thomas Egerton, later Lord Chancellor, with whom she lived until his death in 1617.[3] His oldest son by his previous marriage and his heir, Sir John Egerton, later the first Earl of Bridgewater, in whose honor *Comus* was written, then married Alice's middle daughter Frances. Alice accordingly was both mother-in-law and stepmother to John. The following selective family tree will help to make these complicated inter-relationships clearer, and there are yet more to come.

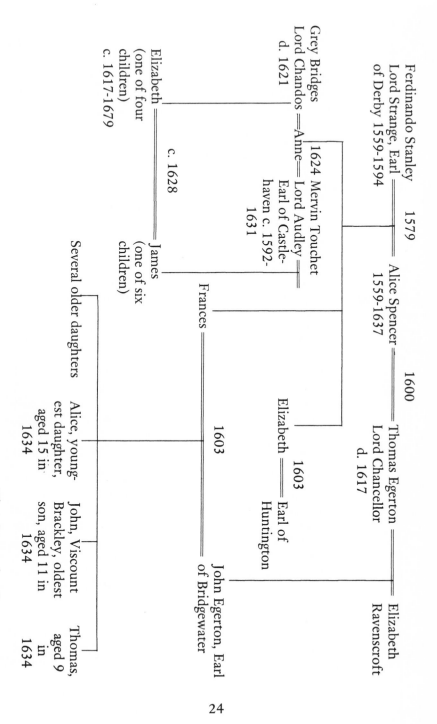

The Actors in *Comus*

Attention now must turn to the tragedy that struck Anne, Alice's oldest daughter. She had been happily married to Grey Bridges, Lord Chandos, until his death in 1621. By him she had four children. As a widow, in 1624 she married Mervin Touchet, Lord Audley and Earl of Castlehaven, a widower also with children. About 1628 he married his oldest child and heir James to Anne's youngest daughter, his step-sister Elizabeth, then aged about eleven. At this point the family history becomes unpleasant—so unpleasant, in fact, that few scholars do more than mention it. Such a thorough biographer as Masson, for example, refers to Anne's marriage only as "a union of unexampled wretchedness"[4] and even our best contemporary biographer, William R. Parker, sees Mervin merely as "infamous," giving no details.[5]

In a study of major importance for an understanding of *Comus*, Barbara Breasted first called attention to the details, information which is easily accessible.[6] What follows here is much indebted to her essay, though there are some additions and some further applications to the interpretation of the play. Specific details about Anne's marital problems are not available until early in 1631, when the married son James brought charges against his father which matched the scandals attached to the murder of Sir Thomas Overbury (Alice's husband had been the trial judge then). In brief, Touchet was charged with having had the two women in his home, his wife Anne and his daughter-in-law Elizabeth, raped, and with practicing sodomy with two servant men of his household. He was tried by twenty-six of his peers who are listed at the beginning of the book reporting the case: *The Arraignment and Conviction of Mervin Lord Audley, Earle of Castlehaven . . . at Westminster, on Monday, April 25, 1631.*[7] His brother-in-law, the Earl of Bridgewater, is not listed as one of these judges, evidently having been excused by the King because of his relationship with the accused.

The details of the testimony are grim indeed. Included in the dramatis personae of this sordid drama, besides Touchet and Anne, and their children James and Elizabeth, is Antill, a former servant married to one of Touchet's daughters. Touchet seems to have planned to disinherit his son James in Antill's favor, plans which may have been the primary cause for the son to bring the charges against him. Other participants were Henry Skipwith, another servant upon whom the lord had bestowed considerable sums of money and other property, a whore named Blandina, resident in the household, who "bestowed an ill disease there,"[8] and two other male servants, Giles Broadway and Lawrence Fitzpatrick.

The trial began with the prosecutor's directing his opening statement to Touchet's treatment of Anne. Having established the principle that any woman, even a whore, may suffer rape, he summarized this part of the case: Touchet's intentions were "to have his wife naught"—that is, prostituted—with Skipworth:

> if she loves him she must love *Henry Skipwith*, whom he loves above all, and not in any honest love, but in a dishonest: he gives his reason by Scripture, she was now subject to him, and therefore if she did ill at his command it was not her fault but his, and he would answer it; he lets this *Skipwith* who he calls his favorite, spend of his purse 500. 1. *per annum*, and if his wife or daughter would have any thing, though necessary, they must lie with *Skipwith* and have it from him, and not otherwise; also telling *Skipwith* and his daughter, that he had rather have a child by him then by any body else.[9]

The record of the testimony then begins. According to Anne's statement before the court,

> The first or second night after we were married, *Antil* came to his bed side whilest we were in bed, and the Lord spake lasciviously to her, and told her, her body was his, and that if she loved him, shee must love *Antil*, and if shee lay with any man with his consent, it was not her fault, but his.

> Hee would make *Skipwith* come naked into her chamber, and bed, and delighted in calling up his servants, making them shew their privities, and her looke on, and commended those that had the largest.

> *Broadway* lay with her whilst she made resistance, and my Lord held her hands, and one of her feet, and she would have killed her self afterwards with a knife, but that hee tooke it from her, and before that act of *Broadway* shee had never done it. He delighted to see the act done, and made *Antil* come into the bed

26

to them, and lye with her whilst he might see it; and that she cryed
out.   (p. 8)

Fitzpatrick corroborated the testimony, stating that

> *Henry Skipwith* was the speciall favourite of the Lord and that he
> usually lay with him; and that *Skipwith* sayd, the Lord made him
> lye with his owne Lady *Awdley,* and that he saw *Skipwith* in his
> sight doe it, my Lord being present, and that he lay with *Blandina*
> in his sight, and foure more, and afterwards he himselfe in their
> sights.   (p. 8)

Skipwith testified to receiving large sums from the Earl, and "He
lay for the most part in bed" with him (p. 8). Mervin also urged
that he have sexual relations with Elizabeth, but he swore that
"she was but thirteene years old when he lay with her, and that
hee could not enter her body without art; and that my Lord gave
her things to open her" (pp. 8-9); other testimony shows that
they were lubricants.

Fitzpatrick then confirmed that the Earl had had intercourse with him, "but did not penetrate his body" (p. 9). The
young Elizabeth offered further confirmation, adding that the
Earl "first tempted [her] to lye with *Skipwith.*" Finally, Broadway testified that he slept in the same room with Mervin and
Anne, and when "in the night he called for Tobacco" and he
brought it, the Earl

> bid him come to bed to him and his wife, and held one of his
> wives legs, and both her hands, and at last he lay with her, not-
> withstanding her resistance.

> That he used his body like a woman. . . .

> He hath seene *Skipwith* and the young Lady lye together in
> bed, and when he got upon her, the Lord hath stood by and en-
> couraged him to get her with childe, and made him kisse his
> Lady, and lye with her, telling him he should not live long, and
> it might be his making.   (pp. 9-10)

One wonders why Fitzpatrick and Broadway were so naive
as to testify as they did, for they were, of course, testifying to

27

to their own guilt as well. After the execution of the Earl on May 14 they too were brought to trial on June 27. It is evident that they thought that the court had promised them leniency for their testimony against the Earl; Broadway "pretended he was promised security from danger, if he would testify against the lord Audley."[10] Anne had to appear again, swearing that her previous evidence was true (p. 419), that Broadway "lay with her by force," and that he had known her carnally and that he did enter her body" (p. 419).

At their public execution at Tyburn on July 16, 1631, Fitzpatrick showed by his prayer that he was a Roman Catholic. He confessed publicly that "his lordship had buggered him, and he his lordship" (p. 422) and that his lordship had incited his attack upon Anne. Broadway too confessed, but to "only lying once with the lady Castlehaven, through persuasion of the Earl, who was then in bed with her; and using some small force for the purpose I did emit, but not penetrate her body" (p. 423). And so they were both hanged, Broadway first and then Fitzpatrick. Presumably it was these public statements which brought the case to public attention, for Charles manged to keep any other report from print until after 1642 when civil war broke out and the record which has been cited appeared, presumably as a piece of propaganda against the nobility.

It is not a pretty story, and one needs little imagination to sense the horror and publicity that it brought to the proud old Countess of Derby and to the Bridgewater family. Quite possibly to show how he sided with them, King Charles almost at once, on June 26, publicly named the Earl to the post of Lord President of Wales, an appointment finally celebrated on the occasion when *Comus* was presented. For his part, Bridgewater seems to have been convinced of his brother-in-law's guilt, for he made no effort to have him pardoned. The execution of a nobleman was not a casual action in those days; because of his rank, however, Touchet was decapitated rather than hanged. He died maintaining his innocence. Near the end of his trial, steadfastly asserting it, he stated.

> that he had nothing more to say, but left himself to God and his peers, and presented to their consideration three woes:

1. Woe to that man, whose Wife should be a Witness against him!

2. Woe to that man, whose Son should prosecute him, and conspire his death!

3. Woe to that man, whose Servants should be allowed Witness to take away his life![11]

Anne's relatives evidently did not believe him. Lady Alice, convinced that her daughter and granddaughter also somehow shared the guilt, spent her time seeking to have the King formally pardon them, which he finally did in November of 1631.[12] She took them both as well as Anne's other children into her home, and they probably participated in *Arcades,* which makes no direct reference to the tragedy but may possibly allude to it as has been suggested above in the discussion of that entertainment. James and Elizabeth were never reconciled; he went on to a notable public career in royalist causes.

As Breasted observes, "it is difficult to believe that *Comus* could have been written and performed with no thought in anyone's mind of how it might allude to the scandal."[13] It had to. In view of the argument already advanced that Milton was carrying out a general directive as to the contents of his masque, it indeed must be assumed that he was responding to commands that he dramatize the virtue of chastity which so many critics have found distasteful. That the family would want to reopen these old wounds seems strange indeed, but the fact is that the performance of *Comus* would certainly recall to the family the events of the spring of 1631 nor could that performance have taken place without their full acceptance of such recognition. It was, however, a delicate subject which Milton was trying to depict, and he may have responded somewhat too enthusiastically; for as been seen the Bridgewater Manuscript omits three important passages which especially stress the issue of chastity (although other obvious sections seem not to have been cut). In any case, there is no evidence that the family were anything except favorable to the Ludlow performance, a strong indication that the centering of the play upon the theme of family virtue ultimately depended upon Bridgewater's directive, strange though we find it that they would want to be reminded of those dreadful times.

It is instructive to see how Milton responded to his commission. In the first place, he certainly turned again to the source which had proved so useful in the composition of *Arcades,* the readings which the Church Calendar directed for September 29.[14] The fact that he did so provides further support, of course, for the argument that he had paraphrased 1 Kings 10 for the entertainment of the previous May. Would the family have attended religious services? Ludlow Castle had its own private chapel, a round Norman building in the inner bailey, presumably with a priest in attendance.[15] According to the epitaph upon his tomb in Little Gaddesden Church at Ashridge, the Earl was "a good Christian,"[16] but even if this were only token praise (and there is no reason to doubt the sincerity of his religious practices) religious rites would assuredly be a part of the solemnities of his installation as Lord President. Accordingly, when Milton turned to the Calendar as he had done earlier in May, he found in the second lesson for Evening Prayer which everyone at Ludlow would have listened to on September 28 the famous statement from 1 Corinthians 13—"Now abideth Faith, Hope, Charity, but the greatest of these is Charity"—which he adapted to the subject had been instructed to undertake, substituting "chastity" for "charity." As in the case of *Arcades,* he could expect the audience to make the immediate association with the reading of the night before.

On the day of the celebration itself, the special holy day of St. Michael and All Angels, Milton found yet further suggesttions in the Lessons directed to be read especially for the occasion. The Evening selection indeed is a reason why September 29 was often chosen for the public celebration of a famous man, as the ceremony at Ludlow was designed to single out the Earl of Bridgewater: it is the forty-fourth chapter of the apocryphal book of Ecclesiasticus, which opens with the well-known verses, "Let us now praise worthy men, and our fathers that begate us. The Lord hath wrought great glory by them. [They are] Such as did beare rule in their kingdomes."

But Milton was even more directly responsive to the reading directed for the Morning Service. A central thesis in the masque is the question of the inherent goodness of nature. Comus argues

30

forcefully that its fecundity which we perceive is meant to be enjoyed:

> Wherefore did Nature powre her bounties forth,
> With such a full and unwithdrawing hand,
> Covering the earth with odours, fruits, and flocks,
> Thronging the Seas with spawne innumerable,
> But all to please, and sate the curious tast? (724-728)

Or, even more directly,

> Beautie is natures coine, must not be hoorded,
> But must be currant, and the good thereof
> Consists in mutual and partaken bliss. (753-755)

Ultimately Comus is arguing from Aristotle's theory of one of the four causes which he thought participate in every existent being (*Physics* 2.7): the final cause. In his view each entity exists to be put to some use, and it does not exist in the fullest sense of the word until it is so employed. The idea has had extensive play in literature; it is, for instance, the Wife of Bath's explanation for putting her "belle chose" to the best use possible. Venus urges the same argument upon the indifferent Adonis in Shakespeare's poem:

> Torches are made to light, jewels to wear,
> Dainties to taste, fresh beauty for the use,
> Herbs for their smell, and sappy plants to bear:
> Things growing to themselves are growth's abuse.
> Seeds spring from seeds, and beauty breedeth beauty;
> Thou wast begot, to get it is thy duty. (163-168)

The concept is inherent in the *carpe diem* poem, but it can also appear in such a profoundly religious one as Gerald Manley Hopkins's "As kingfishers catch fire," which depicts everything as revealing its true nature by what it does; "the just man justices," for example.

As the Lady answers Comus, she cannot deny such evident facts, for Nature's bounty and goodness, including sexuality, are not inherently evil in Protestant eyes and to be repressed. Rather, her response is that the evil pervert Nature to their own evil ends: Nature,

> good cateresse
> Means her provision onely to the good
> That live according to her sober laws
> And holy dictate of spare Temperance. (778-781)

But any of Nature's good things, including sexuality, may be perverted by evil people. In the same way Jesus will refuse Satan's gifts in *Paradise Regained* (2.221), not because they are evil in themselves but because an evil agent has turned them to evil ends.

The subject had already been suggested to Milton and his audience earlier in the religious ceremonies of the day, for it can hardly be a coincidence that the priest read for Morning Prayer on St. Michael's Day Ecclesiasticus 39, which asserts in verses 16 through 27 that

> All the workes of the Lord are exceeding good. . . . A man neede not to say, What is this? wherefore is that? for he hath made all things for their uses. . . . For the good, are good things created from the beginning: so evill things for sinners. The principal things for the whole use of mans life . . . are for good to the godly: so to the sinners they are turned into evil.

Small wonder that Comus is nonplussed:

> She fables not, I feele that I do feare
> Her words set off by some superior power. (814-815)

There was also a special communion service for the day which Milton seems to have studied attentively. For it the priest read Matthew 18, which condemns those who try to incite children to do evil things. According to verse 6, "whoso shall offend one of these little ones which believe in me, it were better for him that a millstone were hanged about his neck, and that he were drowned in the depth of the sea." Here is the original suggestion for the plot of Comus's attack on the children, though Milton makes no suggestion that Comus be drowned.

As he continued to "apt his invention" in Jonson's phrase,

32

Milton turned to the greatest ancient analysis of chastity and virginity, a statement which the family and especially Anne must surely have been directed to reflect upon as they sought comfort for the events of 1631. This is Augustine's *City of God.*

Virginity is a special blessing in the book of Revelation, but members of the early Christian community often suffered rape at the hands of pagans. Augustine found comfort for them in a definition of true chastity as a mental condition which could not be altered by physical assault. As he wrote,

> that power by which man liveth well, resting enthroned, and es-
> tablished in the minde, commands every member of the body,
> and the body is sanctified by the sanctification of the will: which
> sa[n]ctimonie of the will, if it remaine firme and inviolate, what
> way soever the body bee disposed of or abused, (if the partie en-
> during this abuse cannot avoide it without an expresse offence)
> this sufferance layeth no crime upon the soule.[17]

Rape indeed, he goes on, does produce shame—but nothing more: "anothers lust cannot pollute thee." Thus chastity is "a vertue of the minde," not of the body, and "is not lost though the body be violated" (p. 28). This is the "sage/And serious doctrine of Virginitie" (800-801) which Milton had in mind as the classic statement of comfort for the ravished family, and it is this conception which permits the Elder Brother to assert, in opposition to the obvious possibility of rape, that true "Vertue may be assail'd but never hurt" (603).

Augustine's contrasting ideas of force as opposed to acceptance find explicit representation in the two "tools" of Comus's assault: his rod and his cup. It is impossible for anyone not protected by the magic herb haemony to resist the power of his rod (with its phallic suggestions), and this power holds the Lady helpless in her chair regardless of what she wishes: it can "unthred thy joynts/And crumble all they sinewes" (628-629). It fails, however, to subjugate her will to his; for that the content of the cup is necessary as it "unmould[s] reasons mintage" (543); Comus cannot force it upon the mind of his victim as he can the paralyzing power of the rod upon her body. Thus like Augustine's communicants the Lady is physically assailed but guiltless in that she has not concurred with the proposals implied by the cup. The boys destroy it but unaided cannot free their sister from the effects of physical assault. That requires Sabrina's supernatural intervention.

Having adapted Augustine's ideas for the major theme of his masque, Milton evidently found suggestions for further details in the same section of the *City of God.* According to the account in *Comus,* Sabrina, goddess of the Severn River which drains the region of Ludlow, died by drowning herself, a suicide to escape the vengeance of her stepmother. The more usual version of the story which Milton would have known had her thrown into the river by Gwendolen; only in the rather obscure play *Locrine* did she drown herself to avoid capture.[18] In discussing suicide Augustine found that he could excuse if not condone "some holy women . . . in these times of persecution, who . . . threw themselves headlong into a swift river which drowned them and so they died" (p. 39). Unlike Sabrina, their motivation was to save their chastity; and yet like her they represent its holy power.

A final similarity to the *City of God* which Milton may have expected that his audience would recognize is the fact that two scenes of his masque are located in contrasting localities, the Palace of Comus and the Castle of the Bridgewaters at Ludlow. They match the two localities which underlie all of Augustine's book, the City of Man and the City of God. These "two cities (of the predestinate and the reprobate) are in this world" (p. 50) and will remain there until the Last Judgment when they will be separated. Under the guidance of their good Daemon, the children thus escape from the toils of this world to enter the city of God's elect, where they are welcomed by their parents and participate in the climactic dance of the godly which follows. Adulation which figuratively positions the chaste Bridgewaters in the City of God is not unexpected in the Caroline court masque.

So it is that Milton created his play in response to the family directive which itself is somehow a response to the terrible events that reached their crisis in the late spring of 1631. Despite subsequent attacks by many readers, his depiction of the moral issues at the Ludlow performance must have been entirely successful, delicate though the assignment was; the dedication which

Lawes wrote to John Viscount Brackley in 1637 eloquently proves as much. Seen in its family context, Milton's emphasis on chastity can, indeed, receive applause today. But there are yet other elements of family traditions of which Milton was aware and which he wove into the texture of *Comus*. One of them concerns his depiction of the Attendant Spirit, Thyrsis.

NOTES

[1] *The Annales of England* (London, 1605), pp. 767-768.

[2] William Dugdale, *The Baronage of England* (London: 1675), II, 250.

[3] He was later to write of her "cursed railinge and bold tongue," Alix Egerton, *Comus* (1910), p. 14.

[4] I, 591.

[5] II, 759.

[6] "*Comus* and the Castlehaven Scandal," *MS*, 3 (1971), 201-224, which cites a number of manuscript sources besides the two printed texts which are quoted below.

[7] The anonymous *Arraignment* is in the University Microfilms of the Thomason Collection; a second printed record appears in *Cobbett's Complete Collection of State Trials* (London, 1809), III, 408 ff.

[8] *Arraignment*, p. 7.

[9] *Arraignment*, p. 8.

[10] *Cobbett*, p. 421.

[11] *Cobbett*, p. 415.

[12] Breasted gives the details, pp. 215 ff.

[13] Breasted, p. 217.

[14] See also my note, "The Liturgical Context of *Comus*," *ELN,* 10 (1972), 11-15.

[15] Henry John Todd describes the castle at some length in *The Poetical Works of John Milton,* 1st ed. (London, 1801), V, 185-194.

[16] Masson, I, 589.

[17] *The Citie of God,* trans. John Healey (London, 1610), p. 27.

[18] See the summary in the *Variorum Commentary,* II, 957-958.

CHAPTER IV

THE DAEMON IN *COMUS*

The Attendant Spirit in *Comus* whom Milton named Thyrsis originates from a complex background. The name itself derives from the pastoral tradition as that of a shepherd singer in Theocritus 1 and Virgil's Eclogue 7; thus it is another complement to its possessor here, the singer Henry Lawes who was Milton's collaborator. Most obviously, the Spirit is the guardian angel of Christian tradition. But he has a pagan name, he comes to Ludlow from "Before the starry threshold of Jove's court," as he tells the audience in his first line after his opening song, and he returns whence he came. How would the original audience at Ludlow have understood him?

First and most elementary, of course, after his original appearance in an elaborate costume of "skie robes" (97), he announces that henceforth he will disguise himself in the

> weeds and likenesse of a Swaine,
> That to the service of this house belongs   (98-99)

—that is, Henry Lawes will "disguise" himself as Henry Lawes and in a sense will play himself throughout the rest of the masque down to the Epilogue, just as the three children play themselves. He takes care of them too, as he did to some degree in real life.

In the religious rites for the occasion itself Milton found the suggestion for including such a guardian spirit in his play, as he had, as has been shown, for other details. It was staged on the day dedicated to St. Michael and All Angels, the latter viewed,

37

not surprisingly, as guardians. Turning again to the Gospel reading for the communion service which has already been cited once, Matthew 18, one finds in verse 10, "Take heede that yee despise not one of these little ones; for . . . in heaven their angels doe alwayes behold the face of my Father." That means, according to a contemporary interpretation, "God sets his Angels to guard and take speciall charge over those that are least able to defend themselves [and to] Wait for Gods command, to be imployed for the good of poor and humble beleevers." The collect for the service prays for just this salvation: that God may "mercifully graunt that they which alway doe thee service in Heaven, may by thy appointment succour and defend us in earth"—an appropriate plea, as James Taaffe has pointed out, for angelic protection on this particular day.[1] The prayer for such protection repeated in the service of the morning from the gospel reading is answerd by the appearance of Thyrsis in the play staged later in the day.

If such is the origin of the Attendant Spirit in Christian terms, he also seems to have had somewhat more immediate relationships with the Bridgewater family which are revealed implicitly in the texts of the Trinity and Bridgewater Manuscripts, both of which are closer to the performance than is the 1637 edition.[2] In the first stage direction, both manuscripts call Thyrsis not the angel of Christian tradition but a "Guardian spirit, or D(a)emon." Milton seems to have considered that "Daemon" would have a special meaning for the Bridgewater family, for *Dae* continues in the speech headings throughout both manuscripts, but it never appears in the printed forms of 1637 or 1645, which were directed to a wider audience who presumably could not have understood the title in the same sense that the Bridgewaters did.

In classical myth the best-known daemon is probably the one who directed Socrates, according to Plato in the *Apology* and, much elaborated, in the *God of Socrates* by Apuleius. But this daemonic guide is not likely the being that Milton had in mind, for Thyrsis gives positive as well as negative directions to the children, whereas Socrates's daemon told him only what not to do. Milton's comes from "the broad fields of the sky" (4), an area with which the Greek spirit had not been associated. Finally, Augustine views him in the *City of God,* which as has

38

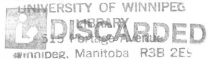

been seen is an important source for ideas in *Comus,* as a dangerous pagan rather than Christian force.[3]

Instead, the primary source of Milton's daemon is Plutarch's *Moralia.* Three of its essays concern the subject: "Why Oracles Cease to Give Answers," "Of the Daemon or Familiar Spirit of Socrates" (which, as has been shown, is of lesser importance), and "Of the Face Appearing in the Moone."[4] But how could Milton assume that the Bridgewaters would recognize his employment of material from these relatively obscure essays?

It seems that Plutarch's daemons had been associated with islands in which the family possessed or had possessed a direct proprietary interest. William Camden opens his description of "The Smaler Ilands in the British Ocean"—the Irish Sea—by citing from "Why Oracles Cease to Give Answers" what Plutarch narrates "generally as touching the Ilands lying neere to Britaine." This material he evaluates as his "First and formost matter." Most of these islands, he says, "lie desert, desolate and scattering heere and there: where of some were dedicated to the *Daemones.*" On a certain one of these, he goes on, "Saturne was by Briareus closed up and kept in prison sound a sleepe (for sleepe was the meanes to hold him captive) about whose person there were many Daemones at his feet that stood attending as servitours." Camden concludes with recognition of the semi-fictional nature of the whole account,[5] but it is clear from the prominent position which he gives the legend as his "First and formost matter" how important he considered the traditional identification of the daemons with islands in the Irish Sea off the coast of Wales.

Plutarch repeats and somewhat enlarges the story in "The Face Appearing in the Moone," identifying Saturn's island now as Homer's Ogygia, home of Calypso, a daughter of Atlas. It is located "distant from great *Britaine* or *England* Westward, five daies sailing." The whole area was called Saturn's sea, and "the giant *Ogygius* or *Briareus*" guards the god there, who sleeps "within the deep cave of a great hollow rock shining and glittering like pure gold." There, "demons or angels doe attend and waite" upon him, and, "having the skill of prophecie and divination, [they] doe of themselves foretell many future things."[6] These same daemons have another home on the moon; from there they come to "act as warders against misdeeds and chastisers of them,"[7] just as Milton's daemon does in *Comus.*

Plutarch located these islands so vaguely that they could have lain almost anywhere west of England (Kepler and others have thought that the passage referred to America).[8]   But from Camden's account quoted above it is quite clear that the earlier seventeenth century English placed them in the Irish Sea—west, that is, of Wales, the domain over which the Earl of Bridgewater was installed as President on September 29, 1634. The two important islands there are Anglesey, just off the northwest coast of Wales, and Man, in the middle of the Irish Sea approximately equidistant from Ireland, Scotland, and Wales—all being visible, as Camden observes, from atop Snaefell, its peak, on a clear day.[9]

Coincidentally, the two islands shared the same name in Latin: "Mona" is Man according to Julius Caesar (*Gallic Wars,* V, 13), but it is Anglesey according to Tacitus (Annals, XIV, 29). In his *History of Britain* Milton expressly follows Tacitus in this identification.[10]   But either of the Monas could fit the legendary site of the sleeping Saturn and his daemonic "serviteurs." ·

The Bridgewaters had strong ties with both islands. Anglesey is, of course, an important part of Wales and thus was a part of the Earl's new responsibilities. As for Man, the family was related to it through Frances and her Derby ancestors. Already mentioned is the fact that the Derbys were the hereditary kings of Man. The claim would have been especially brought home to the family by events at the turn of the century. As has been seen, Ferdinando Stanley died in the spring of 1594. He was succeeded in the title by his brother William. Promptly, according to Dugdale, "a dispute arose betwixt those Heirs Female [the three daughters of Ferdinando and Alice] and him, touching the title to the Isle of Man." The suit, which Dugdale summarizes, ran on for some time and was settled only when the "Earl came to an agreement with those Heirs Female (Daughters to *Ferdinando* Earl of *Derby,* before-mention'd) paying them divers sums of money, to quit their claim thereto: as also with *Thomas* Lord *Ellesmere* (then Lord Chancellour of England [and father of the Earl for whom *Comus* was written]) and *Alice* his wife, widow of the same Earl *Ferdinando.*"[11]   The Derbys and the Bridgewaters, that is, had every reason to claim association with the Isle of Man as well as the more immediate one with Anglesey as part of Wales; Saturn's island could be either of them. Milton seems to have remembered the locality as late as the composition of *Paradise Lost,* which reports that

Saturn old
Fled over *Adria* to th' *Hesperian* Fields,
And ore the *Celtic* roam'd the utmost Isles.   (I, 519-521)

He fled, that is, to England and to the islands west of it that Plutarch had described as his prison.

In *Lycidas* Milton also described the area and its associated mythology three years after *Comus* was staged (indeed, he quite possibly was still revising the earlier play as he began the later poem), for Mona also appears in the elegy: the nymphs protecting the area west of Anglesey when Edward King drowned there were not

on the steep,
Where your old *Bards,* the famous *Druids* ly,
Nor on the shaggy top of Mona high,   (52-53)

a passage in which Milton seems to confuse the two islands, for Man has a mountain, Snaefell, 620 meters high, but little vegetation. Anglesey is flat and fertile—"shaggy." Both had been associated with the Druids. Tacitus, for instance, located them on Anglesey in the same passage cited above in the *History of Britain.* But according to Hector Boece, "Man . . . was sometime the principall seat of the *Druides,*"[12] and in his *History of the Church of Scotland* John Spottiswoode adds under date of 277 A.D. that the Scottish king Cratilinth "made it one of his first works to purge the Kingdome of heathenish superstition, and expelled the *Druids,* a sort of Priests, held in those days in great reputation. [Their] President . . . kept his residence in the Isle of *Man,* [where] they did once every year meet."[13] So Druids were associated with both islands. It seems impossible to decide with finality which of them Milton had in mind as Mona in *Lycidas.* As Allen H. Gilbert remarked long ago, "Milton, who never visited either island, may be giving a composite description."[14] The same uncertainty holds for the island whence

41

Thyrsis comes in *Comus.*

One of the most perplexing passages in *Comus* is its Epilogue, a problem in no way simplified by the fact that the Bridgewater Manuscript shows that Milton had once thought of it as preceding the Daemon's present Prologue. In the printed Epilogue of 1637 and 1645 Thyrsis states that he will now return whence he came: he will fly

> To the Ocean . . .
> And those happy climes that ly
> Where day never shuts his eye,
> Up in the broad fields of the sky.

Carey has shown that the location derives directly from Plutarch: it is the moon, that alternate habitation, as has been seen, of Saturn's attendants, which lies "beyond the range of the earth's shadow" and thus is always in daylight ("Where day never shuts his eye").[15] Carey considers that by the ocean Milton means "the celestial sphere." There Milton locates—and he seems to be unique in this—the Hesperides:

> the Gardens fair
> Of *Hesperus,* and his daughters three
> That sing about the golden tree.

Thus the Epilogue in the printed texts of 1637 and 1645. But the Bridgewater Manuscript puts this material back at the beginning of the play. A likely reason is that Milton originally meant for it to direct the Ludlow audience as to how to recognize quickly the identity of the daemon from information privileged to them (but not to the general reader of the printed texts, which have no such introduction).

According to the Trinity version (closely followed by the printed texts),

> Before the starrie threshold of Joves court
> my mansion is, where those immortal shapes
> of bright aereall spirits live insphear'd
> in regions mild of calme & serene aire.   (1-4)[16]

Such "regions mild of calme & serene aire" seem directly to echo Plutarch's description of Saturn's island: "the nature of the Island and the mildnesse of the aire is wonderfull."[17]   But then continuing in the Trinity Manuscript is material which does not appear in the printed versions of the Prologue: Milton identifies the region with "the Hesperian gardens," an idea which he elaborated in the Bridgewater text and would transfer into the Epilogue.   For the people at the original performance he must have judged that "Hesperian" would for them mean "westward" —the islands, that is, in the Irish Sea already suggested as Saturn's by the "bright aereall spirits" of line 3.   Around this "blisfull Isle," he adds in the Trinity Manuscript alone,

> the jealous ocean that old river winds
> his farre-extended armes till with steepe fall
> halfe his wast flood ye wide Atlantique fills
> & halfe the slow unfadom'd Stygian poole,   (12-15)

a location impossible to identify here with the Moon as Carey does with the material of the Epilogue.   Rather, these lines must refer to an area adjoining the Atlantic and encircling an island in the Irish Sea (the "Stygian poole") west of Ludlow and Wales— "Mona," that is.[18]   Perhaps the family had romanticized their possessions there as the fabled gardens of Hesperus.

In thus alluding to this island west of the audience, a place which he associates with the Hesperides, Milton found a way to identify Thyrsis in terms which the family would understand but with a meaning which seems impossible to recover in full today.   If he did expect them to recognize the allusion, how could he have known in advance that they would do so?   No certain answer now seems possible.   The simplest solution is that there was some kind of tradition in the family of Saturn's association with "their" island and that they thought of it also in terms of the Hesperides.   It had provided them recently with wealth—"golden apples" as it were.   Hesperus's "daughters three" match too the three Derby girls.   Perhaps for some reason the family had recently been reading the *Moralia*.   Whatever the explanation, Lawes would have told Milton that the group could readily recognize the allusion, whereupon it became part of the Prologue.   Later, however, for readers who would not be familiar with the family background, Milton moved this material to the

Epilogue, where it fills a very different function and has, indeed, little conceptual relationship with the masque which now precedes it. In that position he could and did elaborate on the gardens of the Hesperides, which he now moved to the heavens, he deleted the original location between the "Atlantique" and the "Stygian poole" as no longer having any significance; and he added the still-perplexing allusions to Venus and Adonis and to Cupid and Psyche,[19] which had no place in the original performance nor in Plutarch's legend. These gods and demigods have no perceptible relationship with the Bridgewater family and, as the manuscripts show, were not part of Milton's original conception.

Thus it seems that even the Attendant Spirit Thyrsis is something of a domestic, a member of the spirit world associated with the Bridgewater family just as the man who took the part was. The variety of ways in which Milton responded to the family commission is indeed remarkable, his knowledge of the family, its background, and its interests being more extensive and more influential upon *Comus* than has ever been recognized.[20] One would like to know whether he was present at the performance which, as has been seen, was a huge success. Even if he were not there to direct rehearsals, however, it is clear that he so vividly envisioned much of its action that it had to respond in performance to a great many stage directions, actual or implied in his text—the subject last to be considered.

NOTES

[1]*Annotations upon All the Books of the Old and New Testament* (London, 1651, 2nd ed.), *ad* Matt. 18:10 (the fact that the *Annotations* is a Puritan work is a matter of indifference here: Puritans and Anglicans were at one on this passage); James Taaffe, "Michaelmas, the 'Lawless Hour,' and the Occasion of Milton's *Comus*," *ELN*, 6 (1968), 257-262.

[2]For the complex textual problems of *Comus* see John S. Diekhoff,

44

"The Text of *Comus,* 1634 to 1645," *PMLA,* 52 (1937), 705-727, and the articles by John Shawcross cited above as well as Sprott's Introduction.

[3] Pp. 320 ff.

[4] As translated by Philemon Holland, *Morals* (London, 1603). The importance of Plutarch's essays to the masque was first demonstrated by Michael Lloyd, " 'Comus' and Plutarch's Daemons," *N&Q,* 205 (1960), 421-423. Some of his ideas are expanded below. John Carey also used this material to explain certain features of the Spirit's Epilogue in the edition of the minor poems (London, 1960), pp. 225 ff.

[5] *Britain,* pp. 201-202; Holland's translation, p. 1332. For the Greek text and a modern translation see *The Obsolescence of Oracles* in Plutarch, *Moralia,* V, trans. F. A. Babbitt (Loeb Classical Library, 1969), 419E-420A.

[6] Holland's translation, p. 1181.

[7] *The Face on the Moon,* in *Moralia,* XII, trans. Harold Cherniss and William Humbold (Loeb Classical Library, 1969), 944D.

[8] See Babbitt's Introduction in *Moralia* V and W. Hamilton, "The Myth in Plutarch's *De Facie* (940F-945D)," *Classical Quarterly,* 28 (1934), 24 ff.

[9] P. 204.

[10] *Complete Prose Works,* V, i, 75.

[11] *Baronage of England,* II, 250-251.

[12] *The Description of Scotland,* in Raphael Holinshed, *The Chronicles* (London, 1585), Part III, p. 16.

[13] (London, 1655), p. 3. For other early discussions of the Isle of Man see James Chaloner, *A Short Treatise of the Isle of Man,* appended to Daniel King, *The Vale-Royal of England* (London, 1656); and William Sacheverell, *An Account of the Isle of Man* (1702), reprinted in *Publications of the Manx Society,* 1 (1859). Included in the latter is *A Short Dissertation about the Mona of Caesar and Tacitus, the Several Names of Man,* by Thomas Brown.

[14]*A Geographical Dictionary of Milton* (New Haven, 1919), s.v. *Anglesey.*

[15]P. 225, n. 974-975, citing *Moralia* 942F.

[16]From the Scolar facsimile cited above. Cancellations are ignored here and shortened forms are expanded.

[17]Holland, p. 1181.

[18]The *Variorum,* pp. 856-857, notes from B. A. Wright a more mythological interpretation of "Stygian" as related to the nether world: the Ocean feeds both the Styx and the Atlantic.

[19]As John Arthos has observed, "as an allegory the Epilogue is incomplete, [for it] does not work out in an explicitly schematic way the relationship of each of the realms it names. . . . The suggestions are everywhere, the definitions are lacking." "The Realms of Being in the Epilogue of *Comus,*" *MLN,* 76 (1961), 323.

[20]One feature which Milton does not seem to have employed was the Bridgewater coat of arms ("on a chapeau gules turned up ermine, a lion rampant of the first, supporting a broad arrow erect or, headed and feathered argent") and motto ("Sic donec").

CHAPTER V

MILTON'S PRODUCING HAND IN *COMUS*

Although it may seem odd when the fact is pointed out, only John Demaray seems to have considered in detail the performance aspects of *Comus,* and as will appear below he has neglected some of them.[1] Milton has always been more firmly established in the minds of readers as a poet than as a dramatist. Even the professed closet drama *Samson Agonistes* has been performed more frequently. Indeed, there is no way to find out whether he was present at Ludlow on September 29, 1634, or whether he had been within miles of the place during the previous week or so when the performance area there must have been readied for the celebration, the costumes fitted, and time given over to rehearsals. There is no suggestion in the text of *Comus* that he ever visited the castle, as there is in *Arcades* that he had some familiarity with Harefield. His friend and colleague in the production, Henry Lawes, may have overseen everything while Milton stayed at home in Hammersmith with his parents. We simple do not know.

At least since the time of Masson the traditional site of the performance at Ludlow Castle has been its Great Hall, a ruin now for centuries but described by him as "a noble apartment, sixty feet long, thirty wide, and proportionately lofty . . . , the form of which, now roofless and floorless, is still traceable among the ruins."[2] But could this actually have been the location? The square footage is less than one end of a standard basketball court. As French Fogle has pointed out to me in a private communication, "After exploring Ludlow Castle many times, I'm convinced that *Comus* could not have been performed in the Great Hall, which is only 30 x 60 feet, with a great fireplace at one end and a screen at the other to protect the hall from cold winds at the outside entrance. The reduced area would amount to about 30 x 50 at the most, and when you figure ample space for the Earl and his immediate entourage, I just don't see how (1) other notable guests could be accommodated, and (2) there would be enough space for the performance. I think it was performed in the inner bailey, just outside the Great Hall—*pace* almost every critic who has ever written about the actual performance. . . . Only oral tradition puts it in the Great Hall.'' Coincidentally, the bailey is now the location for summer productions of Shakespeare's plays. That Fogle is correct despite the local tradition seems most probable. The acting area absolutely had to possess considerable depth to accommodate the dance of Comus's antimasquers and the discoveries of the three separate scenes, surely one behind the other, which will be described below. Despite the fact that *Comus* was essentially entertainment especially focused upon the family in the audience (and on the stage), that was a numerous family who would be expected to attend. Furthermore, it is difficult to imagine the formal installation of the Lord President of Wales in office without a considerable group of guests, who would later join in the court dances and other festivities of the evening and who would not have been comfortable in the constricted area of the Great Hall. An important corollary to the principle of outdoor performance is that it would necessarily take place before dark; night is conjured up by words and torches as it was upon the public stages.

There is a remarkable amount of evidence that the author had specific actions and effects in mind when he wrote the play, evidence which conclusively proves that he composed the work with the Ludlow performance ever before him, not as a piece of poetry that Lawes could freely adapt to conditions there. Thus it is clear that the singer had told Milton that the two Egerton boys were not sufficiently accomplished singers to be able to perform alone in that mode (the outdoor performance area was perhaps too large for their youthful voices; the Bridgewater Manuscript does show that they may have sung or chanted a few lines along with him to invoke Sabrina, 885 ff.). Milton accordingly assigned no independent music at all to them. The Lady was sufficiently competent for one solo—the Echo Song—which would have support from another singer (Lawes, a contratenor) taking the echo part off stage, but that was to be the limit of her own musical contribution. Lawes seems to have judged that more extensive exhibition of the musical abilities of his pupils on such an important state occasion might run the risk of embarrassing them and their parents. Instead, he left for himself (he was an accomplished singer) all of the songs except the Lady's Echo Song and Sabrina's as she appears.

Beyond such a rather obvious limitation of himself to the performing realities of the participants—and he clearly was told that all three children could handle quite complicated speaking parts, though they may have been shortened for the performance, as the cuts in the Bridgewater Manuscript suggest—Milton reveals his own producing hand in his text with a multitude of directives, express or implied, for the stage business which he envisioned happening at Ludlow. First, of course, and most obvious are the stage directions themselves, minimal indeed by any standards (there are only thirteen in the text read today, and most of them are very brief). But it is surely significant that they are somewhat fuller in the Trinity and Bridgewater Manuscripts, which are closer to the performance, than in the public editions of 1637 and 1645. For instance, instead of the direction, "The Measure," for the antimasque dance at line 145 in the printed texts, the Trinity Manuscript has "the measure (in a wild rude & wanton antick)." At line 161 "they all scatter" in both manuscripts but not in the printed versions, as is true of the direction that "Comus looks in and speaks" at line 278. Presumably the original acting manuscript had as detailed directions as do the Trinity and Bridgewater ones, and perhaps even more. But as the performance moved further and further into the past, Milton realized that readers would approach his text more as poetry on the page than as stage action and so reduced them to the barest minimum when the play appeared in print.

Such stage directions as do survive show at times that their author was uncertain of just how the effects that he wanted might be achieved. In the first one, according to the Bridgewater text, "a guardian spiritt or demon descends or enters" (Trinity omits the last three words but the printed texts retain them), suggesting that Milton was not present at rehearsals or performance to know whether there was stage machinery at Ludlow which would permit the perfomer to be lowered gracefully to the stage as could happen in the Great Hall or whether he merely walked on outdoors in the bailey. An attractive idea is that for the latter he came from the round Norman chapel, which is well placed in the inner bailey for the performance. The Epilogue at the end of the Trinity Manuscript directs that "The Daemon sings or says" it as he prepares to fly or run from the stage, Milton apparently being unaware of just how it was performed at Ludlow. The direction "sings or says" disappears in both printed texts, where the Spriit merely "Epiloguizes"—a statement that only a reader would need to know. As a matter of fact, Lawes set at least part of the Epilogue to music, which survives. For another change, as Sabrina descends, having released the Lady, Thyrsis must have sung lines 936-951, for at line 951 both Bridgewater and Trinity direct, "Song ends;" there is no suggestion in 1637 or 1645 that it was anything but spoken.

On the other hand, Milton also wrote some firm stage directions which he evidently meant to be followed. For the beginning of his play, he stated, "The first scene discovers a wild wood," which is directed in all the early texts. A fact sometimes overlooked is that "scene" for Milton here meant in modern terms "scenery." As the OED states (I.6), a scene is "the material apparatus, consisting chiefly of painted hangings, slides, etc., set at the back and sides of the stage," adding that such "painted scenes . . . were a principal feature of the privately produced masques of Jas. I and Chas. I." Thus for Milton's first "scene" a curtain was raised or drawn aside to reveal painted scenery representing "a wild wood." The second scene, again discovered—this time when the scenery of the wild wood is removed from before it (and the stage is empty of actors)—is of the exterior, not the interior, of Comus's palace, as Demaray and others have remarked.[3] Placed before it are a table set "with all dainties" and the Lady seated in a chair. The third and final discovery (again with no actors on stage) reveals the scenery, also exterior, of Ludlow and its castle; the audience would be expected to recognize the contrast of palace and castle as paralleling Augustine's cities of man and God. Such practical stage effects are entirely typical of the Stuart masque though they are rather simpler than most, perhaps in view of the lack of suitable machinery at Ludlow as compared with that which was available in London. Directions for lighting effects, so important for some of Jonson's scenes, are implied rather than expressly given, as will appear below.

It must be admitted, however, that for one action Milton's staging is quite unclear in a modern reconstruction. This is the point where "Sabrina rises, attended by water-Nymphs, and sings" at line 903. At the end of her scene she "descends." Obviously she appears to the audience, accompanied by several other ladies, but how was it done? The two manuscripts are of no help here. Because Sabrina sings that her "sliding Chariot stays" for her "By the rush-fringed bank," most critics have assumed that this group rises on some sort of platform, perhaps a sled or wagon, ornamented to look like a chariot with agates, turkis, and emeralds as the following lines describe it, pulled on rising tracks up on to the stage where it stops before the painting of Comus's palace (this is still the "scene"). Sabrina steps off and walks, singing, to where the Lady is restrained in her chair. Such staging is spectacular and dramatically effective in the masque tradition.

On the other hand, such a chariot-sled would be awkward to handle, it would have to be large enough to accommodate several singing women, and it would be heavy in proportion. If indeed it rises any distance at all it would require application of a good deal of force to move and lift it as well as a good deal of back-stage space where it could be mounted. Much simpler is to have Sabrina and her accompanying nymphs merely appear as they mount stairs at the side of the stage (probably not the back, where the next scene, at Ludlow, is being readied). It would be even more effective outdoors in the bailey if she and her companions were to appear from the Chapel. As she "rises" in this manner, Sabrina sings of her dwelling place, the river, which she depicts as a "sliding Chariot," an interpretation urged by Brooks and Hardy.[4]   Her description of the blue and green ornaments then is to be understood as applied to the sparkling water in the river, supposed to be behind her, as

> from off the waters fleet
> Thus I set my printless feet
> O're the Cowslips Velvet head   (910-912)

to approach the Lady. In the same way, Thyrsis's song as she descends applies to the water of the Severn. Such staging is far simpler than the presentation of an actual vehicle, but Milton's directions are not sufficiently clear that his original intentions

51

can be reconstructed with certainty. In view of the isolation of Ludlow the simpler arrangements seem more practical. One fact which the technical devices required by Milton suggest is that he himself may have witnessed one or more court masques, though how or under what circumstances it is impossible to guess today. But even though he titled his work "Maske," the fact that critics have had difficulty fitting the work into the genre suggests that his familiarity was not profound. Milton's inexperience in writing for the stage is further evidenced by the fact that he found it necessary to repeat the long exposition of Comus's background (60-91) through the mouth of Thyrsis in an awkward and dull recapitulation when he meets the boys (534-554) and then to recapitulate the song which opened the play, the intrusion of Comus's antimasquers, and the Lady's echo song—all of which the audience has seen—in Thyrsis's narrative of the incidents (557-581). It seems likely that Lawes, who had certainly participated in the production of masques, actively collaborated with Milton but only on practical problems of staging.

Such are the suggestions from the surviving stage directions about how Milton envisioned his play for the actual performance. But even more interesting are the actions which the dialogue required to be made. They show vividly just how Milton was able to visualize in advance an actual performance and to control it through his text. Other dramatists do the same thing. When Shakespare, for instance, writes, "But soft! what light through yonder window breaks?," Juliet simply must appear above, illuminated in some way at a window (it is "night"), whether or not there is a stage direction in the original text to say so (there is none). It is remarkable how thoroughly Milton mastered this technique in *Comus.* He must have attended many plays and attentively studied the techniques which they employed.[5]

Thus, what did he intend to happen as the curtain rose to reveal the "dark wood"? When he first meets the two brothers Thyrsis reports that earlier that evening he had been enjoying his own music: he

began
Wrapt in a pleasing fit of melancholy
To meditate my rural minstrelsie,

(559-561)

when a noise of riot broke out "At which I ceas't, and listen'd them a while." Here Milton gives a late description of what had happened as the performance began: probably after some kind of musical overture, Lawes as the Daemon entered singing. And, indeed, in the Bridgewater Manuscript as has been seen, the performance began with a song of fourteen lines, "From the Heavns now I fly," which in all the other versions appears in somewhat altered form at the beginning of the Epilogue. Then Thyrsis spoke, giving the exposition which is interrupted by the racket of Comus and his followers, who enter at line 106. Meanwhile, Thyrsis has described in lines 84 ff. what they must look like when they appear. Textual critics have for the most part assumed that Milton originally wrote "From the Heavns now I fly" for the Epilogue and then moved it to the Prologue, but lines 559-561 argue for the reverse procedure and that when he placed the passage later he neglected to change these lines, which still report them as beginning the play.

At line 45 Milton directs that Lawes indicate the man whom the occasion was celebrating—"A noble peer of mickle trust and power," the Earl of Bridgewater—by bowing to him where he was seated in the hall and describing the importance of his investiture that day. At line 97 he requires that upon his first appearance the Attendant Spirit be dressed in some appropriate "daemonic" costume—his "skie robes." Finally, he tells the audience (and the actor) that when he next appears he will be "disguised" as himself—as Henry Lawes, that is—who "to the service of this house belongs," as has already been seen. As he concludes his long speech, "I must be viewless now," Milton directs that he exit.

When the three children appear, they too are dressed in their own clothes to "play" themselves, possibly a unique arrangement in the history of English drama though not really alien to the spirit of the masque tradition. It simplified the movement from illusion to reality when the Attendant Spirit, as Lawes, presented them to their parents in the audience at the close of their performance. And it reinforced the idea of an attack upon the chastity and virtue of a member of the family—an attack now successfully resisted (as had been true only in Augustine's sense three years earlier).

Some of Milton's implied stage directions are sufficiently

obvious to require no more than passing comment. According to line 182 Comus must step aside into concealment, though he stays on stage, as the Lady enters. Milton imagined that the stage itself would be relatively dark, for in her next speech she hopes for some light in the darkness of the wood:

> Was I deceav'd, or did a sable cloud
> Turn forth her silver lining on the night? (235-236)

Sure enough, someone high up on the set opened a dark lantern so that she can at once exclaim,

> I did not err, there does a sable cloud
> Turn forth her silver lining on the night. (237-238)

At line 279 the dialogue requires that Comus come forward to speak to her. At line 344 she must follow him off stage ("Shepheard lead on"), just as at line 672 the boys follow Thyrsis off. The audience would be expected to recognize the parallel actions and the allegorical contrast, the girl unconsciously following the bad shepherd, the boys the good one. At line 494 there must be an off-stage halloo, repeated at line 500 just before Thyrsis enters to the boys (and they briefly draw their swords until they learn his identity; the Trinity Manuscript indeed directs that both calls be given). Comus's lines 814-820 must be spoken as an aside; Sabrina must sprinkle drops upon the Lady's breast (925) and three times each on her fingers and lips before she touches the chair in which the Lady is magically bound (930-932). Such directions are quite obviously implied by the dialogue. A neat trick on Milton's part is his arrangement that the magic drug haemony need never be actually visible to the audience: Thyrsis has "purs't it up" (656) and so he need not show it as he describes it; he promises to give it later to the boys "when wee goe" (662). When they attack Comus later they need not be encumbered with it nor wear it visibly.

Some directions that Milton gives his actors, however, are clothed in various degrees of obscurity. One of the simpler requirements is that Comus must

> hurle
> My dazling Spells into the spungie aire (167-168)

54

—that is, he tosses up some kind of "magic" dust which will sparkle in the light and delude the Lady into seeing him as "som harmles Villager," and he probably repeats the action at line 179. This obviates his having to change his costume before he meets her, and as has been seen he does not exit to do so; he merely steps aside. The audience continues to see him visibly as an enchanter, but she supposedly cannot.

Especially interesting are the tableaux which she says that she can see at line 230 and which must be visible to the audience: "O welcome pure-ey'd Faith," she declares, "white-handed Hope . . . , And thou unblemish't forme of Chastity," all of whom, she adds, she can see "visibly." Milton is directing that they appear somewhere at the back of the stage at that moment in a sudden illumination, made visible both to her and to the attentive audience, the bright tableaux contrasting with the yet-dark stage where she is "lost." As has been mentioned, these lines do not appear in the Bridgewater Manuscript, though they are in both the Trinity one and in the 1637 edition. Some have argued that they are cut because of their overly strong affirmation of Faith, Hope, and Chastity, but I do not agree. The passage begins by stressing the fact that it is a dark, starless night; the Lady wanders in "single darkness" before the virtues suddenly appear to her "visibly." On an outdoor stage in daylight such tableaux as Milton imagines her seeing would be quite ineffective in comparison with an indoor performance which he must have originally had in mind and in which they could be suddenly, miraculously revealed by artificial lighting. For the same reason the deletion continues so as to include those lines where the Lady sees "a sable cloud/Turn forth her silver lining on the night," an effect likewise impossible for a daylight performance. Thus it seems likely that this entire passage was in Milton's original text, written for indoors, and was cut (by Lawes?) because of the different conditions of outdoor performance rather than because of its strong moral contents.

Somewhat more obscurely, Thyrsis must come silently on stage at about line 291 during the stichomythic passage between the Lady and Comus, and leave at about its end, hidden from the other actors but in view of the audience; for he later tells the two brothers at lines 584-591 that he had "found the place" where the Lady and Comus were talking but he reports only that part of the conversation there. "Longer I durst not stay," he adds, and so he fled. One may even speculate that, when the Brothers rush in with their swords drawn to save their sister, Comus and his company may seem to emit smoke as they "make sign of resistance," for Thyrsis warns that they will pretend to fight back and may "like the sons of *Vulcan* vomit smoake" (669), a spectacular bit of business indeed if the producer could pull it off.

Although the stage direction at line 827 has the boys "wrest his Glass out of his hand, and break it against the ground," it is silent about the "charming rod" with its phallic implications which Comus carried in his other hand. Thyrsis had been concerned most of all that it be seized (line 667) and is dismayed at their failure to do so, for the Lady must consequently remain physically powerless. In his emphasis upon possession of this rod Milton may have had in mind the association of the name *Thyrsis* with *thyrsus,* the name for the ivy-twined wand which Bacchus traditionally bore and hence the source of Comus's. It is necessary, the Spirit says, that "his rod" be "revers'd" (line 830) if the Lady is to be freed from her silent enchantment in the chair. In terms of the play upon Thyrsis/thyrsus, that is, the power which the wand represents is a natural one which has been misused and thus must be reversed (but not destroyed as the glass was), the same point that the Lady had made against Comus a few lines earlier in her rejection of his argument from nature as favoring fertility in any guise. Thyrsis thus represents a power of nature in its sexual but chaste guise, Comus's thyrsus its reversal. Natural sexuality, that is, is good; its depravity is not. As many critics have observed, in *Comus* Milton is not denying sexuality—a proper part of nature and of life—but its reversal, its unnatural misuse.

To conclude upon somewhat more certain ground this discussion of how Milton envisioned the staging of *Comus,* the masque dances proper follow line 989, having been introduced as a

> victorious dance
> O're sensual folly, and intemperance,

though one can only imagine the stately form they would take, without the "duck or nod" of the peasant dance at line 971 or the bacchanal of Comus and his rout earlier. Such courtly activities end with the re-entrance of the Spirit to sing his final piece at the next line.

But between line 989 and 990 one must imagine a considerable gap of time, perhaps as much as several hours. Both manuscripts direct, "The dances *all* end" (emphasis added). Jonson regularly allows for such an interval in his masques during which the audience would disperse to various entertainments such as dancing and dining. Shakespeare introduces similar interruptions in some of his plays written for courtly presentations. In *The Tempest,* a work often thought to have influenced *Comus,* the masque occupied most of the short Act IV, to be followed in Act V by the reconciliation of the several issues. But between IV and V in the court performance there seems to have been a break, perhaps a rather long one.[6] An even better illustration can be found in the conclusion to *A Midsummer Night's Dream.* There, the "lamentable comedy" of Pyramus and Thisbe being completed, Bottom asks Theseus whether he wants to "see the epilogue, or to hear a Burgomask dance." The king emphatically chooses the latter, rejecting the epilogue, and a dance accordingly follows. But then there is an epilogue after all which Theseus himself delivers. Everyone leaves the stage. Then Puck unexpectedly enters to reintroduce Oberon and Titania, accompanied by fairies, who deliver yet a second epilogue and go out. Finally, Puck alone has yet a third epilogue, a soliloquy of fourteen lines. Such a set of epilogues is quite perplexing and can best be understood if one allows a long gap of time between Theseus's exit and Puck's entrance (the third epilogue, it is generally agreed, is directed to a different audience).[7] Modern productions which attempt to play Act 5 straight through to the end always find this part of the last act impossible to do in a convincing fashion, a bad afterthought or anti-climax, for presentation of both endings seriatim makes no sense at all. They must have been very effective when separated by some time in the original performance. If, as has been argued, *Comus* was presented outdoors in the bailey, everyone at this point may well have moved indoors to the Great Hall for the rest of the evening.

From a masque by John Marston, already mentioned, which had been written expressly in 1607 at the direction of her daughter, the Countess of Huntington, to honor Lady Alice, Todd cites for "the curious and liberal reader" just such an extended interval as must have taken place at Ludlow. During the final song.

> the Masquers presented theire sheelds, and tooke forth their Ladyes to daunce.

> After they hadd daunced many measures, galliards, corantos, and lavaltos, the night being much spent; whilst the Masquers prepared themselves for theire departing measure,

Cynthea, the "presenter," came back on stage to speak an eighteen-line epilogue.[8]   In just the same way, and like Puck, Milton's Attendant Spirit enters at the proper time as determined by the Earl.   Having clothed himself once again in his "sky robes,"[9] Thyrsis ends the evening with his departure, pronouncing as he goes a moral benediction, so to speak, on all of the audience present and reiterating the theme of the masque which the Bridgewaters wanted so much to be affirmed:

> Love virtue, she alone is free
> She can teach you how to clime
> Higher than the sphery chime;
> Or if Virtue feeble were,
> Heavn'n itself would stoop to her

in the purificatory rites for the family on that evening long ago.

NOTES

[1] *Milton and the Masque Tradition* (Cambridge, Massachusetts, 1968), Chapter V: "Staging *Comus* at Ludlow."   Several of the interpretations of this book are incorporated here, sometimes with modifications.   For a tabu-

lation of all of the stage directions from the manuscripts and printed texts see Shawcross, ''Certain Relationships,'' pp. 54-56.

[2] I, 610.

[3] Demaray, pp. 101-102, 104, 116-117, and *Variorum,* p. 967.

[4] Cleanth Brooks and J. E. Hardy, *Poems of Mr. John Milton* (New York, 1951), p. 225; *Variorum,* p. 967.

[5] The stage directions implied in Shakespeare's texts have, of course, been spelled out in more or less detail by every editor since Rowe. For an example of how they enlighten certain plays see the unpublished doctoral dissertation of Barbara Hodgdon, ''The Look of the Play: Dramatic Forces in Shakespeare's Early History Plays'' (University of New Hampshire, 1974).

[6] See E. Law, ''Shakespeare's *Tempest* as originally produced at Court,'' *English Association Pamphlet* (1920).

[7] See the argument in the Appendix for these original conditions.

[8] V, 153. Eliot quotes the conclusion of this masque in the epigraphs to his ''Burbank with a Baedeker'': ''now the countess [that is, Lady Alice] passed on until she came through the little park, where Niobe presented her with a cabinet, and so departed.''

[9] Demaray thinks that he resumes this dress earlier, when he presents the children to their parents, but this seems questionable: Milton would have him ''disguised'' as a man during all of his intercourse with human beings in the play.

CHAPTER VI

A TENTATIVE PROMPTBOOK FOR *COMUS*

In 1637 when Henry Lawes, presumably with Milton's assistance and approval, prepared the text of *Comus* for the press, the evening at Ludlow was almost three years past. Unlike plays, masques were never revived after an initial performance or rarely two. Thus it is not surprising that the 1637 text emphasized its poetry rather than its dramatic aspects, which are minimally described. When in 1645 Milton included the play in the first collection of his poetry with the public acknowledgement that he was its author, the distance was even greater. The letter from Sir Henry Wotton commending it which Milton printed then stresses the "delicacy itself" of its "Songs and Odes, whereunto I must plainly confess to have seen nothing parallel in our Language." It was offered, that is, as poetry to its readers rather than as drama; and so it has for the most part remained.

And yet, as has been seen, the work takes on a new vitality when one makes the effort to reconstruct the circumstances at Ludlow Castle on September 29, 1634. The text which follows attempts to illustrate this by recreating what seem to have been Milton's original intentions that Lawes would carry out. The results of this approach provide a text unlike any other, including the two manuscripts and the printed forms of 1637 and 1645. Because all four of them are readily available (the first three most conveniently in Sprott's edition already mentioned), it seems legitimate to take such freedom with the text here as staging it would suggest. Those familiar with the play may be surprised by the presence of the opening song and even dismayed by the greatly curtailed Epilogue. But, as has been argued above, such seem to have been Milton's original intentions.

The text which follows is rearranged from that of 1637, its major disagreements with the Bridgewater Manuscript indicated in the footnotes. There are no references here to the other manuscript, the Trinity, because they would be hopelessly confusing and in any case would add no more information about the performance than does the Bridgewater. Although the speeches are those of 1637 (its few misprints silently corrected), the stage directions are those of Bridgewater except in the few places where the two are substantially the same. Contractions in these directions are silently expanded and all are italicized (as they were not in the original) to separate them clearly from the text which they accompany. All newly added stage directions are also italicized and are in brackets to distinguish them from Milton's. In a few places punctuation has been modernized. For his speech headings I have used the manuscript *Dae(mon)* for the *Spir(it)* of the printed texts.

The music which Lawes composed for five of the songs survives in several manuscripts. Other music, like that which Sabrina sang, has disappeared, possibly because its composer did not care to preserve it. These surviving pieces have been edited from British Museum Additional Manuscript 11518. The Lady's Echo Song was performed with an echoing voice (Lawes) answering her from offstage or with an instrumental response. The musical effect may be achieved in a number of ways; I suggest here one for the first phrase of the composition. A full arrangement for piano and voice of all the songs is in Andrew J. Sabol, *Songs and Dances for the Stuart Masque* (Providence, Rhode Island, 1959).

If, as I have argued, the play was performed outdoors in the castle bailey, it would take place late in the afternoon or early in the evening, before dark. This may be the reason why lines 202-204 were also cut in the Bridgewater Manuscript:

> They left me then, when the gray-hooded Ev'n
> Like a sad Votarist in Palmers weeds
> Rose from the hindmost wheels of *Phoebus* waine

because it was not dark during the performance. There could thus be no artificial lighting; only Comus's "route" carry torches to reinforce the idea of night. The actors could have access to the stage through doors or windows of the Great Hall, before which the performances would take place.

One may only guess at most of the costuming. The Daemon originally enters in "sky clothes"—probably blue, perhaps with rainbow hues—which he then changes to become Henry Lawes and assumes again for his final song. The boys may well have had on the masquing clothes which they had worn the previous spring when they participated in Thomas Carew's masque *Coelum Britannicum.* Surely the Lady would be dressed in white; it seems likely that the seductive Comus would be in red (the blue of the Daemon, white of the Lady, and red of Comus being the three primary colors recognized then as John Donne observes in his *First Anniversary,* line 361). The grotesquely headed monsters are easy enough to imagine. Sabrina, of course, must have been clothed and ornamented with symbols to suggest her river home, as must her attendants. It seems unlikely that any of the actors would wear masks unless Comus himself did. And maybe Sabrina.

After the main curtain is drawn back, the Daemon enters a scene representing a dark wood, mostly conveyed by a painted back drop. This then too is drawn aside to "discover" the exterior of Comus's palace, where the Lady is sitting in a chair before a table covered with food. Finally, this is drawn aside to "discover" the last scene, a depiction of the town of Ludlow and its dominant castle where the play is taking place. Or was scenery simply discarded here, the "scene" being the outside of the castle itself? The dance of the monsters and the second one of the peasants need not be in the staging area: they could more freely take place on the ground of the bailey. Finally, when Thyrsis presents the children to their parents, he merely leads them, as he sings, from the staging area directly to where John and Frances are sitting prominently in the audience.

A MASKE

*[After a musical introduc-
tion,] The first sceane discovers a wild wood, then a
guardian spiritt or demon
descendes or enters [, singing:]*

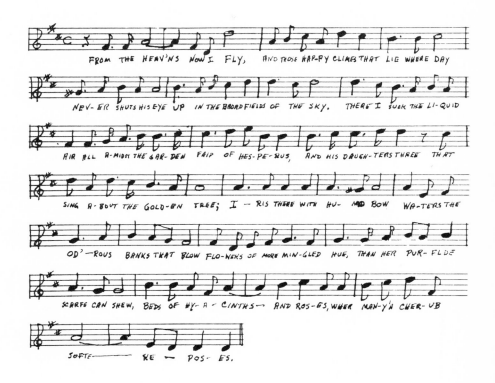

FROM THE HEAV'NS NOW I FLY, AND THOSE HAP-PY CLIMES THAT LIE WHERE DAY

NEV-ER SHUTS HIS EYE UP IN THE BROAD FIELDS OF THE SKY. THERE I SUCK THE LI-QUID

AIR ALL A-MIDST THE GAR-DEN FAIR OF HES-PE-RUS, AND HIS DAUGH-TERS THREE THAT

SING A-BOUT THE GOLD-EN TREE; I — RIS THERE WITH HU- MID BOW WA-TERS THE

OD'—ROUS BANKS THAT BLOW FLO-WERS OF MORE MIN-GLED HUE, THAN HER PUR-FLDE

SCARFE CAN SHEW, BEDS OF HY-A-CINTHS— AND ROS-ES, WHER MAN-Y'A CHER-UB

SOFTE— RE — POS-ES.

Before the starrie threshold of *Joves* Court
My mansion is, where those immortall shapes
Of bright aëreall Spirits live insphear'd
In Regions mild of calme and serene aire,
Above the smoake and stirre of this dim spot
20 Which men call Earth, and with low-thoughted care
Confin'd, and pester'd in this pin-fold here,
Strive to keepe up a fraile, and feaverish being
Unmindfull of the crowne that Vertue gives
After this mortall change to her true Servants
Amongst the enthron'd gods on Sainted seats.
Yet some there be that by due steps aspire
To lay their just hands on that golden key
That ope's the palace of Aeternity:
To such my errand is, and but for such
30 I would not soile these pure ambrosial weeds
With the ranck vapours of this Sin-worne mould.
　　　But to my task. *Neptune* besides the sway
Of every salt Flood, and each ebbing Streame
Tooke in by lot 'twixt high, and neather *Jove*
Imperial rule of all the Sea-girt Iles
That like to rich, and various gemms inlay
The unadorned bosome of the Deepe,
Which he to grace his tributarie gods
By course commits to severall government
40 And gives them leave to weare their Saphire crowns,
And weild their little tridents, but this Ile
The greatest, and the best of all the maine
He quarters to his blu-hair'd deities,
And all this tract that fronts the falling Sun　　　*[Indicating the*
A noble Peere of mickle trust, and power　　　*Earl in the*
Has in his charge, with temper'd awe to guide　　　*Audience.]*
An old, and haughtie Nation proud in Armes:
Where his faire off-spring nurs't in Princely lore
Are comming to attend their Fathers state,
50 And new-entrusted Scepter, but their way
Lies through the perplex't paths of this dreare wood,
The nodding horror of whose shadie brows
Threats the forlorne and wandring Passinger.
And here their tender age might suffer perill

But that by quick command from Soveraigne *Jove*
I was dispatcht for their defence, and guard,
And listen why, for I will tell yee now
What never yet was heard in Tale or Song
From old, or moderne Bard in hall, or bowre.

60   *Bacchus* that first from out the purple Grape
Crush't the sweet poyson of mis-used Wine
After the *Tuscan* Mariners transform'd
Coasting, the *Tyrrhene* shore, as the winds listed,
On *Circes* Iland fell (who knows not *Circe*
The daughter of the Sun? whose charmed Cup
Whoever tasted lost his upright shape,
And downward fell into a grovling Swine).
This Nymph that gaz'd upon his clustring locks
With Ivie berries wreath'd, and his blith youth

70   Had by him, ere he parted thence, a Son
Much like his Father, but his Mother more,
Whom therefore she brought up and *Comus* nam'd,
Who ripe, and frolick of his full growne age
Roaving the *Celtick,* and *Iberian* fields
At last betakes him to this ominous wood,
And in thick shelter of black shades imbowr'd
Excells his Mother at her mightie Art,
Offring to every wearie Travailer
His orient liquor in a Chrystall glasse

80   To quench the drouth of *Phoebus,* which as they tast
(For most doe tast through fond intemperate thirst)
Soone as the Potion works, their humane count'nance
Th'expresse resemblance of the gods is chang'd
Into some brutish forme of Wolfe, or Beare
Or Ounce, or Tiger, Hog, or bearded Goat,
All other parts remaining as they were,
And they, so perfect is their miserie,
Not once perceive their foule disfigurement,
But boast themselves more comely then before

90   And all their friends and native home forget,
To roule with pleasure in a sensuall stie.
Therefore when any favour'd of high *Jove*
Chances to passe through this adventrous glade,
Swift as the Sparkle of a glancing Starre
I shoote from heav'n to give him safe convoy,
As now I doe: but first I must put off

66

These my skie robes spun out of *Iris* wooffe,
And take the weeds and likenesse of a Swaine,
That to the service of this house belongs,
100   Who with his soft Pipe, and smooth-dittied Song,
Well knows to still the wild winds when they roare,
And hush the waving woods, nor of lesse faith,
And in this office of his Mountaine watch,
Likeliest, and neerest to the present aide
Of this occasion. But I heare the tread
Of hatefull steps, I must be viewlesse nowe.   *Exit*

> Comus *enters with a*
> *charminge rod in one hand*
> *& a glass of liquor in the*
> *other[;] with him a route of*
> *monsters like men & women*
> *but headed like wild*
> *beasts[;] their apparell glist-*
> *ringe, they come in makinge*
> *a riotous and unruely noise*
> *with torches in their hands.*

    Comus. The starre that bids the Shepheard fold,
Now the top of heav'n doth hold,
And the gilded Carre of Day
110   His glowing Axle doth allay,
In the steepe *Atlantik* streame,
And the slope Sun his upward beame
Shoots against the duskie Pole,
Pacing toward the other gole
Of his Chamber in the East.
Meane while welcome Joy, and Feast,
Midnight shout, and revelrie,
Tipsie dance, and Jollitie.
Braid your Locks with rosie Twine,
120   Dropping odours, dropping Wine.
Rigor now is gone to bed,
And Advice with scrupulous head,
Strict Age, and sowre Severitie
With their grave Sawes in slumber lie.
We that are of purer fire,
Immitate the starrie quire,

Who in their nightly watchfull Spheares,
Lead in swift round the Months and Yeares.
The Sounds, and Seas with all their finnie drove,
130 Now to the Moone in wavering Morrice move,
And on the tawny sands and shelves,
Trip the pert Fairies and the dapper Elves;
By dimpled Brooke, and Fountaine brim,
The Wood-nymphs deckt with daisies trim,
Their merry wakes, and pastimes keepe,
What hath night to doe with sleepe?
Night hath better sweets to prove,
Venus now wakes, and wakens Love.
Come let us our rights begin
140 'Tis onely day-light that makes Sin
Which these dun shades will ne're report.
Haile Goddesse of Nocturnall sport
Dark-valid *Cotytto,* t'whom the secret flame
Of mid-night Torches burnes; mysterious Dame
That ne're art call'd, but when the Dragon woome
Of Stygian darknesse spets her thickest gloome
And makes one blot of all the aire,
Stay thy clowdie *Ebon* chaire,
Wherein thou rid'st with *Hecat',* and befriend
150 Us thy vow'd Priests, till utmost end
Of all thy dues be done, and none left out
Ere the blabbing Easterne scout
The nice Morne on th'*Indian* steepe
From her cabin'd loop hole peepe,
And to the tel-tale Sun discry
Our conceal'd Solemnity.
Come, knit hands, and beate the ground
In a light fantastick round.

[They dance] The measure
in a wild, rude, & wanton
Antick [until Comus inter-
rupts:]

Break off, breake off, I feele the different pace
160 Of some chast footing neere about this ground.
Run to your shrouds, within these Brakes, and Trees   *they all*
Our number may affright: Some Virgin sure   *scatter*

68

(For so I can distinguish by mine Art)
Benighted in these woods. Now to my charmes
And to my wilie trains; I shall e're long
Be well stock't with as faire a Heard as graz'd
About My Mother *Circe*. Thus I hurle   *[Tosses sparkling*
My dazling Spells into the spungie aire   *dust into the air.]*
Of power to cheate the eye with bleare illusion,
170   And give it false presentments, lest the place
And my queint habits breed astonishment,
And put the Damsel to suspicious flight,
Which must not be, for that's against my course;
I under faire praetents of friendly ends,
And wel plac't words of glozing courtesie
Baited with reasons not unplausible
Wind me into the easie hearted man,
And hug him into snares; when once her eye
Hath met the vertue of this Magick dust,   *[Tosses dust again.]*
180   I shall appeare some harmless Villager
Whom thrift keepes up about his Country geare.
But here she comes. I fairly step aside   *[Hides.]*
And hearken, if I may, her buisnesse here.

The Ladie enters.

This way the noise was, if mine eare be true
My best guide now, me thought it was the sound
Of Riot, and ill manag'd Merriment,
Such as the jocond Flute, or gamesome Pipe
Stirs up among the loose unleter'd Hinds
When for their teeming Flocks, and granges full
190   In wanton dance they praise the bounteous *Pan*,
And thanke the gods amisse. I should be loath
To meet the rudeness, and swill'd insolence
Of such late Wassailers; yet ô where else
Shall I informe my unacquainted feet
In the blind mazes of this tangled wood?
My Brothers when they saw me wearied out
With this long way, resolving here to lodge
Under the spreading favour of these Pines
Stept as they se'd to the next Thicket side
200   To bring me Berries, or such cooling fruit
As the kind hospitable woods provide.

They left me then, when the gray-hooded Ev'n[1]
Like a sad Votarist in Palmers weeds
Rose from the hindmost wheels of *Phoebus* waine.
But where they are, and why they came not back
Is now the labour of my thoughts, 'tis likeliest
They had ingag'd their wandring steps too far,
And envious darknesse, e're they could returne,
Hold stolne them from me,[2] else ô theevish Night
210   Why shouldst thou, but for some fellonious end
In thy darke lanterne thus close up the Stars,
That nature hung in Heav'n, and fill'd their lamps
With everlasting oile to give due light
To the misled, and lonely Travailer.
This is the place, as well as I may guesse
Whence even now the tumult of loud Mirth
Was rife, and perfect in my listening eare,
Yet nought but single darknesse doe I find.
What might this be? a thousand fantasies
220   Begin to throng into my memorie
Of calling shapes, and beckning shadows dire,
And ayrie tongues, that syllable mens names
On Sands, and Shoars, and desert Wildernesses.
These thoughts may startle well, but not astound
The vertuous mind, that ever walks attended
By a strong siding champion Conscience.
O welcome pure-ey'd Faith, white-handed Hope   *[Tableaux ap-*
Thou flittering Angel girt with golden wings,   *pear of the three*
And thou unblemish't forme of Chastitie   *Virtues illuminated.]*
230   I see yee visibly, and now beleeve
That he, the Supreme good, t'whom all things ill
Are but a slavish officers of vengeance
Would send a glistring Guardian if need were
To keepe my life, and honour unassail'd.
Was I deceiv'd, or did a sable cloud
Turne forth her silver lining on the night?

*[A dark lantern opens above
to simulate the moon shining through clouds.]*

---

[1] Lines 202-204 are not in *BM*.

[2] From here through line 239 are not in *BM*.

I did not erre, there does a sable cloud
Turne forth her silver lining on the night
And casts a gleame over this tufted Grove.

240   I cannot hallow to my Brothers, but
Such noise as I can make to be heard fardest
Ile venter, for my new enliv'nd spirits
Prompt me; and they perhaps are not farre off.

[She sings, being answered by an echo offstage.]

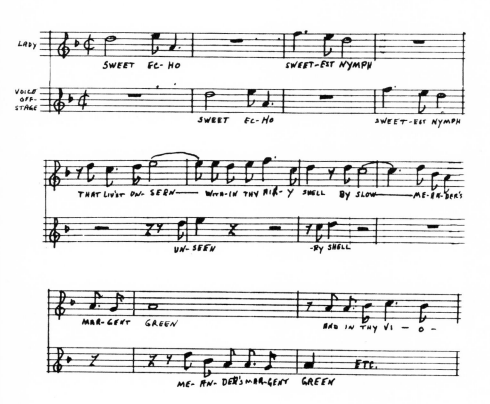

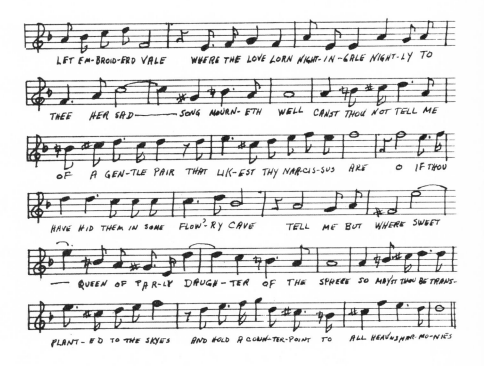

LET EM-BROID-ERD VALE WHERE THE LOVE LORN NIGHT-IN-GALE NIGHT-LY TO

THEE HER SAD———SONG MOURN-ETH WELL CANST THOU NOT TELL ME

OF A GEN-TLE PAIR THAT LIK-EST THY NAR-CIS-SUS ARE O IF THOU

HAVE HID THEM IN SOME FLOW²-RY CAVE TELL ME BUT WHERE SWEET

— QUEEN OF PAR-LY DAUGH-TER OF THE SPHERE SO MAYST THOU BE TRANS-

PLANT-ED TO THE SKYES AND HOLD A COUN-TER-POINT TO ALL HEAVNS HAR-MO-NIES

Comus Looks in [i.e., appears] & Speaks

   Com. Can any mortall mixture of Earths mould
   Breath such Divine inchanting ravishment?
260 Sure something holy lodges in that brest,
   And with these raptures moves the vocal aire
   To testifie his hidden residence;
   How sweetly did they float upon the wings
   Of Silence, through the emptie-vaulted night
   At every fall smoothing the Raven downe
   Of darknesse till she smil'd: I have oft heard
   My mother *Circe* with the Sirens three
   Amidst the flowrie-kirtl'd *Naiades*
   Culling their Potent hearbs, and balefull drugs
270 Who as they sung, would take the prison'd soule
   And lap it in *Elysium, Scylla* wept,

And chid her barking waves into attention,
And fell *Charybdis* murmur'd soft applause:
Yet they in pleasing slumber lull'd the sense
And in sweet madnesse rob'd it of it selfe,
But such a sacred, and home-felt delight,
Such sober certainty of waking blisse
I never heard till now. Ile speake to her
And she shall be my Queene. Haile forreine wonder

[steps forward]

280 Whom certaine these rough shades did never breed
Unless the Goddesse that in rurall shrine
Dwell'st here with *Pan*, or *Silvan*, by blest Song
Forbidding every bleake unkindly Fog
To touch the prosperous growth of this tall wood.
 La. Nay gentle Shepherd ill is lost that praise
That is addrest to unattending Eares,
Not any boast of skill, but extreame shift
How to regaine my sever'd companie
Compell'd me to awake the courteous Echo
290 To give me answer from her mossie Couch.
 Co. What chance good Ladie hath bereft you thus?

     [Enter Thyrsis silently at rear.]

 La. Dim darknesse, and this leavie Labyrinth.
 Co. Could that divide you from neere-ushering guides?
 La. They left me weary on a grassie terfe.
 Co. By falshood, or discourtesie, or why?
 La. To seeke i'th vally some coole friendly Spring.
 Co. And left your faire side all unguarded Ladie?
 La. They were but twain, & purpos'd quick return.
 Co. Perhaps fore-stalling night praevented them.
300 *La.* How easiè my misfortune is to hit!
 Co. Imports their losse, beside the praesent need?
 La. No lesse then if I should my brothers lose.
 Co. Were they of manly prime, or youthful bloom?
 La. As smooth as *Hebe's* their unrazord lips.
 Co. Two such I saw, what time the labour'd Oxe
In his loose traces from the furrow came,
And the swink't hedger at his Supper sate;
I saw them under a greene mantling vine
That crawls along the side of yon small hill,
310 Plucking ripe clusters from the tender shoots,
Their port was more than humaine; as they stood,

73

I tooke it for a faërie vision
Of some gay creatures of the element
That in the colours of the Rainbow live
And play i'th plighted clouds, I was aw-strooke,
And as I past, I worshipt; if those you seeke   *[Exit Thyrsis.]*
It were a journy like the path to heav'n
To helpe you find them.
    La. Gentle villager
What readiest way would bring me to that place?
320   *Co.* Due west it rises from this shrubbie point.
    La. To find out that good shepheard I suppose
In such a scant allowance of starre light
Would overtask the best land-pilots art
Without the sure guesse of well-practiz'd feet.
    Co. I know each lane, and every alley greene
Dingle, or bushie dell of this wild wood,
And every boskie bourne from side to side
My daylie walks and ancient neighbourhood,
And if your stray attendance be yet lodg'd
330 Or shroud within these limits, I shall know
Ere morrow wake, or the low-roosted larke
From her thach't palate rowse, if otherwise
I can conduct you Ladie to a low
But loyall cottage, where you may be safe
Till further quest.
    La. Shepheard I take thy word,
And trust thy honest offer'd courtesie,
Which oft is sooner found in lowly sheds
With smoakie rafters, then in tapstrie halls,
And courts of Princes, where it first was nam'd,
340 And yet is most praetended: in a place
Lesse warranted then this, or lesse secure
I cannot be, that I should feare to change it.
Eye me blest Providence, and square my triall
To my proportion'd strength. Shepheard lead on.   *[Exeunt.]*

[Enter] The two Brothers.

    Eld. bro. Unmuffle yee faint stars, and thou fair moon
That wontst to love the travailers benizon
Stoope thy pale visage through an amber cloud
And disinherit *Chaos,* that raigns here

74

In double night of darknesse, and of shades;
350 Or if your influence be quite damm'd up
With black usurping mists, some gentle taper
Though a rush candle from the wicker hole
Of some clay habitation visit us
With thy long levell'd rule of streaming light
And thou shalt be our starre of *Arcadie*
Or *Tyrian* Cynosure.

     2 Bro. Or if our eyes
Be barr'd that happinesse, might we but heare
The folded flocks pen'd in their watled cotes,
Or sound of pastoral reed with oaten stops,
360 Or whistle from the Lodge, or village cock
Count the night watches to his featherie Dames,
T'would be some solace yet, some little chearing
In this close dungeon of innumerous bowes.
But ô that haplesse virgin our lost sister
Where may she wander now, whether betake her
From the chill dew, amongst rude burs and thistles?
Perhaps some cold banke is her boulster now
Or 'gainst the rugged barke of some broad Elme
Leans her unpillow'd head fraught with sad fears.
370 What if in wild amazement, and affright
Or while we speake within the direfull graspe
Of Savage hunger, or of Savage heat?[3]

     Eld. bro. Peace brother, be not over exquisite
To cast the fashion of uncertaine evils,
For grant they be so, while they rest unknowne
What need a man forestall his date of griefe
And run to meet what he would most avoid?
Or if they be but false alarms of Feare
How bitter is such selfe-delusion?
380 I doe not thinke my sister so to seeke
Or so unprincipl'd in vertues book

---

[3] For lines 370-379 *BM* substitutes:
    or els in wild amazement and affright,
    soe fares as did forsaken *Proserpine*
    when the bigg rowling flakes of pitchie clouds
    and darkness wound her in.

And the sweet peace that goodnesse bosoms ever
As that the single want of light, and noise
(Not being in danger, as I trust she is not)
Could stir the constant mood of her calme thoughts
And put them into mis-becomming plight.
Vertue could see to doe what vertue would
By her owne radiant light, though Sun and Moon
Were in the flat Sea sunck, and Wisdoms selfe
390   Oft seeks to sweet retired Solitude
Where with her best nurse Contemplation
She plumes her feathers, and lets grow her wings
That in the various bustle of resort
Were all to ruffl'd, and sometimes impair'd.
He that has light within his owne cleere brest
May sit i'th center, and enjoy bright day,
But he that hides a darke soule, and foule thoughts
Benighted walks under the mid-day Sun,
Himselfe is his owne dungeon.
         2 Bro. 'Tis most true
400   That musing meditation most affects
The Pensive secrecie of desert cell
Farre from the cheerefull haunt of men, and heards,
And sits as safe as in a Senat house,
For who would rob an Hermit of his weeds
His few books, or his beades, or maple dish,
Or doe his gray hairs any violence?
But beautie like the faire Hesperian tree
Laden with blooming gold, had need the guard
Of dragon watch with uninchanted eye
410   To save her blossoms, and defend her fruit
From the rash hand of bold Incontinence.
You may as well spread out the unsun'd heaps
Of misers treasure by an outlaws den
And tell me it is safe, as bid me hope
Danger will winke on opportunitie
And let a single helplesse mayden passe
Uninjur'd in this wild surrounding wast.
Of night, or lonelynesse it rocks me not,
I feare the dred events that dog them both,
420   Lest some ill greeting touch attempt the person
Of our unowned sister.
         Eld. Bro. I doe not brother

76

Inferre, as if I thought my sisters state
Secure without all doubt, or controversie:[4]
Yet where an equall poise of hope, and feare
Does arbitrate th'event, my nature is
That I encline to hope, rather then feare
And gladly banish squint suspicion.
My sister is not so defencelesse left
As you imagine, she has a hidden strength
430 Which you remember not.
   2 Bro. What hidden strength
Unlesse the strength of heav'n, if you meane that?
   Eld. Bro. I meane that too, but yet a hidden strength
Which if heav'n gave it, may be term'd her owne:
'Tis chastitie, my brother, chastitie:
She that has that, is clad in compleate steele,
And like a quiver'd nymph with arrowes keene
May trace huge forrests, and unharbour'd heaths,
Infamous hills, and sandie perillous wilds
Where through the sacred rays of chastitie
440 No savage fierce, bandite, or mountaneere
Will dare to soyle her virgin puritie,
Yea there, where very desolation dwells
By grots, and caverns shag'd with horrid shades[5]
She may passe on with unblench't majestie
Be it not done in pride, or in presumption.
Some say no evill thing that walks by night
In fog, or fire, by lake, or moorish fen
Blew meager hag, or stubborne unlayd ghost
That breaks his magicke chaines at curfeu time

---

[4] For line 423 *BM* substitutes:
 secure, without all doubt or question, no;
 I could be willinge though now i'th darke to trie
 a tough encounter, with the shaggiest ruffian
 that lurks by hedge or lane, of this dead circuit
 to have her by my side, though I were suer
 she might be free from perill where she is,

[5] *BM* adds:
 and yawnings denns, where glaringe monsters house

450 No goblin, or swart Faërie of the mine
Has hurtfull power ore true virginity.
Doe yee beleeve me yet, or shall I call
Antiquity from the old schools of Greece
To testifie the armes of Chastitie?
Hence had the huntresse *Dian* her dred bow,
Faire silver-shafted Queene for ever chast,
Wherewith she tam'd the brinded lionesse
And spotted mountaine pard, but set at nought
The frivolous bolt of *Cupid;* gods and men
460 Fear'd her sterne frowne, & she as queen oth' woods.
What was that snakie headed *Gorgon* sheild
That wise *Minerva* wore, unconquer'd virgin
Wherewith she freez'd her foes to congeal'd stone?
But rigid looks of Chast austeritie
And noble grace that dash't brute violence
With sudden adoration, and blancke aw.
So deare to heav'n is saintly chastitie
That when a soule is found sincerely so,
A thousand liveried angels lackie her,
470 Driving farre off each thing of sinne, and guilt,
And in cleere dreame, and solemne vision
Tell her of things that no grosse eare can heare,
Till oft converse with heav'nly habitants
Begin to cast a beame on th' outward shape,
The unpolluted temple of the mind,
And turnes it by degrees to the souls essence
Till all bee made immortall; but when lust
By unchast looks, loose gestures, and foule talke
But most by leud, and lavish act of sin
480 Lest in defilement to the inward parts,
The soule growes clotted by contagion,
Imbodies, and imbrutes, till she quite loose
The divine propertie of her first being.
Such are those thick, and gloomie shadows damp
Oft seene in Charnell vaults, and Sepulchers
Hovering, and sitting by a new made grave
As loath to leave the body that it lov'd,
And link't it selfe by carnall sensualitie
To a degenerate and degraded state.
490 *2 Bro.* How charming is divine Philosophie!
Not harsh, and crabbed as dull fools suppose,

78

But musicall as is *Apollo's* lute,
And a perpetuall feast of nectar'd sweets
Where no crude surfet raigns.
    Eld. bro. List, list I heare   *[Offstage call.]*
Some farre off hallow breake the silent aire.
    2 Bro. Me thought so too, what should it be?
    Eld. Bro. For certaine
Either some one like us night founder'd here,
Or else some neighbour wood man, or at worst
Some roaving robber calling to his fellows.

500   *2 Bro.* Heav'n keepe my sister, agen, agen, and neere,
                           [Call again.]
Best draw, and stand upon our guard.   *[Brothers draw swords.]*
    Eld. bro. Ile hallow,
If he be friendly he comes well, if not
Defence is a good cause, and Heav'n be for us.

                                 he hallows and is answered,
                                 the guardian daemon comes
                                 in habited like a shepheard.

That hallow I should know, what are you, speake,
Come not too neere, you fall on iron stakes else.
    Dae. What voice is that, my yong Lord? speak agen.
    2 Bro. O brother 'tis my fathers Shepheard sure.
    Eld. bro. Thyrsis? whose artfull strains have oft delayd
The huddling brook to heare his madrigale,

510   And sweeten'd every muskrose of the dale,
How cam'st thou here good Swaine, hath any ram
Slip't from the fold, or yong kid lost his dam,
Or straggling weather the pen't flock forsook?
How couldst thou find this darke sequester'd nook?
    Dae. O my lov'd masters heire, and his next joy,
I came not here on such a triviall toy
As a strayed Ewe, or to pursue the stealth
Of pilfering wolfe; not all the fleecie wealth
That doth enrich these downs is worth a thought

520   To this my errand, and the care it brought.
But ô my virgin Ladie where is she,
How chance she is not in your companie?
    Eld. bro. To tell thee sadly shepheard, without blame
Or our neglect, wee lost her as wee came.

Dae. Aye me unhappie then my fears are true.

Eld. bro. What fears good *Thyrsis?* prethee briefly shew.

Dae. Ile tell you, 'tis not vaine, or fabulous
(Though so esteem'd by shallow ignorance)
What the sage Poëts taught by th'heav'nly Muse
530 Storied of old in high immortall verse
Of dire *Chimera's* and inchanted Iles
And rifted rocks whose entrance leads to hell,
For such there be, but unbeliefe is blind.
Within the navill of this hideous wood
Immur'd in cypresse shades a Sorcerer dwells
Of *Bacchus,* and of *Circe* borne, great *Comus.*
Deepe skill'd in all his mothers witcheries,
And here to every thirstie wanderer
By slie enticement gives his banefull cup
540 With many murmurs mixt, whose pleasing poison
The visage quite transforms of him that drinks,
And the inglorious likeness of a beast
Fixes instead, unmoulding reasons mintage
Character'd in the face; this have I learn't
Tending my flocks hard by i'th hilly crofts
That brow his bottome glade, whence night by night
He and his monstrous rout are heard to howle
Like stabl'd wolves, or tigers at their prey
Doing abhorred rites to *Hecate*
550 In their obscured haunts of inmost bowres.
Yet have they many baits, and guilefull spells
T'inveigle, and invite th'unwarie sense
Of them that passe unweeting by the way.
This evening late by then the chewing flocks
Had ta'ne their supper on the savourie herbe
Of Knot-grass dew-besprent, and were in fold
I sate me downe to watch upon a bank
With ivie canopied, and interwove
With flaunting hony-suckle, and began
560 Wrapt in a pleasing fit of melancholy
To mediate my rural minstrelsie
Till fancie had her fill, but ere a close
The wonted roare was up amidst the woods,
And filld the aire with barbarous dissonance
At which I ceas't, and listen'd them a while
Till an unusuall stop of sudden silence

Gave respit to the drowsie frighted steeds
That draw the litter of close-curtain'd sleepe.
At last a soft, and solemne breathing sound
570   Rose like a steame of rich distill'd Perfumes
And stole upon the aire, that even Silence
Was tooke e're she was ware, and wish't she might
Deny her nature, and he never more
Still to be so displac't. I was all eare,
And took in strains that might create a soule
Under the ribs of Death, but ô ere long
Too well I did perceive it was the voice
Of my most honour'd Lady your deare sister.
Amaz'd I stood, harrow'd with griefe and feare,
580   And ô poore haplesse nightingale thought I,
How sweet thou sing'st, how neere the deadly snare!
Then downe the lawns I ran with headlong hast
Through paths, and turnings often trod by day
Till guided by mine eare I found the place
Where that dam'd wisard hid in slie disguise
(For so by certain signs I knew) had met
Alreadie, ere my best speed could praevent
The aidlesse innocent Ladie his wish't prey,
Who gently ask't if he had seene such two,
590   Supposing him some neighbour villager;
Longer I durst not stay, but soone I guess't
Yee were the two she mean't; with that I sprung
Into swift flight till I had found you here,
But farther know I not.

     2 Bro. O night and shades
How are yee joyn'd with hell in triple knot
Against th'unarmed weaknesse of one virgin
Alone, and helplesse! is this the confidence
You gave me brother?

     Eld. bro. Yes, and keep it still,
Leane on it safely, not a period
600   Shall be unsaid for me; against the threats
Of malice or of sorcerie, or that power
Which erring men call Chance, this I hold firme,
Vertue may be assail'd, but never hurt,
Surpriz'd by unjust force, but not enthrall'd,
Yea even that which mischiefe meant most harme,
Shall in the happie triall prove most glorie.

But evill on it selfe shall backe recoyle
And mixe no more with goodnesse, when at last
Gather'd like scum, and setl'd to it selfe
610 It shall bee in eternall restlesse change
Selfe fed, and selfe consum'd; if this faile
The pillar'd firmament is rottennesse,
And earths base built on stubble. But come let's on.
Against th'opposing will and arme of heav'n
May never this just sword be lifted up,
But for that damn'd magician, let him be girt
With all the greisly legions that troope
Under the sootie flag of *Acheron,*
Harpyies and *Hydra's,* or all the monstrous bugs
620 'Twixt *Africa,* and *Inde,* Ile find him out
And force him to restore his purchase backe
Or drag him by the curles, and cleave his scalpe
Downe to the hipps.
  Dae. Alas good ventrous youth,
I love thy courage yet, and bold Emprise,
But here thy sword can doe thee little stead:
Farre other arms, and other wapons must
Be those that quell the might of hellish charms:
He with his bare wand can unthred thy joynts
And crumble all thy sinewes.
  Eld. Bro. Why prethee shepheard
630 How durst thou then thy selfe approach so nëere
As to make this relation?
  Dae. Care and utmost shifts
How to secure the Ladie from surprisall
Brought to my mind a certaine shepheard lad
Of small regard to see to, yet well skill'd
In every vertuous plant, and healing herbe
That spreds her verdant leafe to th'morning ray.
He lov'd me well, and oft would beg me sing,
Which when I did, he on the tender grasse
Would sit, and hearken even to extasie,
640 And in requitall ope his leather'n scrip,
And shew me simples of a thousand names
Telling their strange, and vigorous faculties.
Amongst the rest a small unsightly root,
But of divine effect, he cull'd me out;
The leafe was darkish, and had prickles on it,

But in another Countrie, as he said,
Bore a bright golden flowre, but not in this soyle:
Unknowne, and like esteem'd, and the dull swayne
Treads on it dayly with his clouted shoone,
650   And yet more med'cinall is it then that *Moly*
That *Hermes* once to wise *Ulysses* gave.[6]
He call'd it *Haemony,* and gave it me
And bad me keepe it as of soveraine use
'Gainst all inchantments, mildew blast, or damp
Or gastly furies apparition;
I purs't it up, but little reck'ning made
Till now that this extremity compell'd,
But now I find it true, for by this means
I knew the foule inchanter though disguis'd,
660   Enter'd the very limetwigs of his spells,
And yet came off: if you have this about you
(As I will give you when wee goe) you may
Boldly assault the necromancers hall,
Where if he be, with dauntlesse hardihood
And brandish't blade rush on him, breake his glasse,
And shed the lushious liquor on the ground,
But sease his wand, though he and his curst crew
Feirce signe of battaile make, and menace high,
Or like the sons of *Vulcan* vomit smoake,
670   Yet will they soone retire, if he but shrinke.
     Eld. Bro. Thyrsis lead on apace. Ile follow thee,
And some good angell beare a sheild before us.

                  [Exeunt, Thyrsis leading.]

               *The Scene Changes to a
stately palace set out with
all manner of deliciousnesse,
soft musicke, tables spred
with all dainties.* Comus *ap-
peares with his rabble, and
the Ladie set in an inchanted chaire to whom he offers*

---

[6] Lines 646-651 are not in *BM.*

 Comus. Nay Ladie sit; if I but wave this wand,
Your nervs are all chain'd up in alablaster,
And you a statue; or as *Daphne* was
Root bound that fled *Apollo.*
 La. Foole doe not boast:
Thou canst not touch the freedome of my mind
With all thy charms, although this corporall rind
Thou hast immanacl'd, while heav'n sees good.
680 *Co.* Why are you vext Ladie, why doe you frowne?
Here dwell no frowns, nor anger, from these gates
Sorrow flies farre: see here be all the pleasurs
That fancie can beget on youthfull thoughts
When the fresh blood grows lively, and returns
Brisk as the *April* buds in primrose season.
And first behold this cordial julep here
That flames, and dances in his crystall bounds
With spirits of balme, and fragrant syrops mixt.
Not that *Nepenthes* which the wife of *Thone*
690 In *Aegypt* gave to *Jove*-borne *Helena*
Is of such power to stirre up joy as this,
To life so friendly, or so coole to thirst.
Why should you be so cruell to your selfe,
And to those daintie limms which nature lent
For gentle usage, and soft delicacie?
But you invert the cov'nants of her trust,
And harshly deale like an ill borrower
With that which you receiv'd on other termes,
Scorning the unexempt condition,
700 By which all mortall frailty must subsist,
Refreshment after toile, ease after paine,[7]
That have been tir'd all day without repast,
And timely rest have wanted, but faire virgin
This will restore all soone.
 La. T'will not false traitor,

---

[7] For lines 693-701 *BM* reads:
 poore ladie thou hast neede of some refreshinge

84

T'will not restore the truth and honestie
That thou hast banish't from thy tongue with lies.
Was this the cottage, and the safe abode
Thou told'st me of? what grim aspects are these,
These ougly-headed monsters? Mercie guard me!
710   Hence with thy brewd inchantments, foule deceiver,
Hast thou betray'd my credulous innocence
With visor'd falshood, and base forgerie,
And wouldst thou seek againe to trap me here
With lickerish baits fit to ensnare a brute?[8]
Were it a draft for *Juno* when she banquets
I would not tast thy treasonous offer; none
But such as are good men can give good things,
And that which is not good, is not delicious
To a wel-govern'd and wise appetite.
720   *Co.* O foolishnesse of men! that lend their eares
To those budge doctors of the *Stoick* furre,
And fetch their praecepts from the *Cynick* tub,
Praising the leane, and sallow Abstinence.
Wherefore did Nature powre her bounties forth
With such a full and unwithdrawing hand,
Covering the earth with odours, fruits, and flocks,
Thronging the seas with spawne innumerable
But all to please, and sate the curious tast?
And set to work millions of spinning worms,
730   That in their green shops weave the smooth-hair'd silk
To deck her Sons, and that no corner might
Be vacant of her plentie, in her owne loyns
She hutch't th'all worshipt ore, and precious gems
To store her children with; if all the world
Should in a pet of temperance feed on Pulse,
Drink the clear streame, and nothing weare but Freize,
Th'all-giver would be unthank't, would be unprais'd,
Not halfe his riches known, and yet despis'd,
And we should serve him as a grudging master,
740   As a penurious niggard of his wealth,
And live like Natures bastards, not her sons,
Who would be quite surcharg'd with her own weight,

---

[8] *BM* lacks lines 711-714.

And strangl'd with her wast fertilitie;
Th'earth cumber'd, and the wing'd aire dark't with plumes
The heards would over-multitude their Lords,
The sea ore-fraught would swell, and th'unsought diamonds
Would so emblaze the forehead of the Deep,
And so bestudde with stars that they below
Would grow inur'd to light, and come at last
750   To gaze upon the Sun with shameless brows.
List Ladie, be not coy, and be not cosen'd
With that same vaunted name Virginitie:
Beautie is natures coine, must not be hoorded,
But must be currant, and the good thereof
Consists in mutuall and partaken blisse,
Unsavourie in th'injoyment of it selfe.
If you let slip time, like a neglected rose
It withers on the stalke with languish't head.
Beautie is natures brag, and must be showne
760   In courts, at feasts, and high solemnities
Where most may wonder at the workmanship;
It is for homely features to keepe home,
They had their name thence; course complexions
And cheeks of sorrie graine will serve to ply
The sampler, and to teize the huswifes wooll.
What need a vermeil-tinctur'd lip for that,
Love-darting eyes, or tresses like the Morne?
There was another meaning in these gifts,
Thinke what, and be adviz'd, you are but yong yet.[9]
770   *La.* I had not thought to have unlockt my lips
In this unhallow'd aire, but that this Jugler
Would thinke to charme my judgement, as mine eyes
Obtruding false rules pranckt in reasons garbe.
I hate when vice can bolt her arguments
And vertue has no tongue to check her pride:
Impostor, doe not charge most innocent nature
As if she would her children should be riotous
With her abundance; she good cateresse
Means her provision only to the good
780   That live according to her sober laws

---

[9] *BM* lacks lines 751-769.

And holy dictate of spare temperance.
If every just man that now pines with want
Had but a moderate, and beseeming share
Of that which lewdly-pamper'd Luxurie
Now heaps upon some few with vast excesse,
Natures full blessings would be well dispenc't
In unsuperfluous even proportion,
And she no whit encomber'd with her store,
And then the giver would be better thank't,
790   His praise due paid, for swinish gluttony
Ne're looks to heav'n amidst his gorgeous feast,
But with besotted base ingratitude
Cramms, and blasphemes his feeder. Shall I goe on?
Or have I said enough? to him that dares
Arme his profane tongue with reproachfull words
Against the Sun-clad power of Chastitie
Faine would I something say, yet to what end?
Thou hast nor Eare, nor Soule to apprehend
The sublime notion, and high mysterie
800   That must be utter'd to unfold the sage
And serious doctrine of Virginitie,
And thou art worthy that thou shouldst now know
More hapinesse then this thy praesent lot.
Enjoy your deere Wit, and gay Rhetorick
That hath so well beene taught her dazling fence,
Thou art not fit to heare thy selfe convinc't;
Yet should I trie, the uncontrouled worth
Of this pure cause would kindle my rap't spirits
To such a flame of sacred vehemence,
810   That dumb things would be mov'd to sympathize,
And the brute Earth would lend her nerves, and shake,
Till all thy magick structures rear'd so high
Were shatter'd into leaps ore thy false head.

    Co. She fables not, I feele that I doe feare   *[Aside.]*
Her words set off by some superior power;
And though not mortall, yet a cold shuddring dew
Dips me all o're, as when the wrath of *Jove*
Speaks thunder, and the chaines of *Erebus*
To some of *Saturns* crew. I must dissemble,

87

820 And try her yet more strongly.[10] Come; no more, *[Again aloud.]*
This is meere morall babble, and direct
Against the canon laws of our foundation.
I must not suffer this, yet 'tis but the lees
And setlings of a melancholy blood;
But this will cure all streight, one sip of this   *[Offering the*
Will bathe the drooping spirits in delight   *cup again.]*
Beyond the blisse of dreams. Be wise, and tast.

> *The brothers rushe in with*
> *swords drawne, wrest his*
> *glasse of liquor out of his*
> *hand, and breake it against*
> *the ground[;] his rowte*
> *make signe of resistance,*
> *[seeming to breathe out*
> *smoke; Comus waves his*
> *wand over the lady to para-*
> *lyze her], but [all] are all*
> *driven in; the Demon is to*
> *come in with the brothers.*

Dae. What, have you let the false enchanter scape?
O yee mistooke, yee should have snatcht his wand
830 And bound him fast; without his rod revers't,
And backward mutters of dissevering power
Wee cannot free the Ladie that sits here
In stonie fetters fixt, and motionlesse;
Yet stay, be not disturb'd, now I bethinke me,
Some other meanes I have which may be us'd,
Which once of *Melibaeus* old I learnt,
The soothest shepheard that ere pipe't on plains.
There is a gentle nymph not farre from hence
That with moist curb sways the smooth Severn stream,
840 *Sabrina* is her name, a virgin pure,
Whilome shee was the daughter of *Locrine,*
That had the scepter from his father *Brute.*
She guiltlesse damsell flying the mad pursuit

---

[10]*BM* lacks from "feeder," line 793, through "strongly," line 820.

Of her enraged stepdam *Guendolen*
Commended her faire innocence to the flood
That stay'd her flight with his crosse-flowing course,
The water Nymphs that in the bottome playd
Held up their pearled wrists and tooke her in,
Bearing her straite to aged *Nereus* hall
850 Who piteous of her woes reard her lanke head,
And gave her to his daughters to imbathe
In nectar'd lavers strewd with asphodil,
And through the porch, and inlet of each sense
Dropt in ambrosial oyles till she reviv'd,
And underwent a quicke, immortall change
Made goddesse of the river; still she retaines
Her maiden gentlenesse, and oft at eve
Visits the heards along the twilight meadows,
Helping all urchin blasts, and ill lucke signes
860 That the shrewd medling elfe delights to make,
Which she with precious viold liquors heales,
For which the shepheards at their festivalls
Carroll her goodnesse lowd in rusticke layes,
And throw sweet garland wreaths into her streame
Of pancies, pinks, and gaudie daffadills.
And, as the old Swaine said, she can unlocke
The clasping charme, and thaw the numming spell,
If she be right invok't in warbled Song,
For maidenhood she loves, and will be swift
870 To aid a virgin such as was her selfe
In hard besetting need; this will I trie
And adde the power of some adjuring verse.   [*Sings:*]

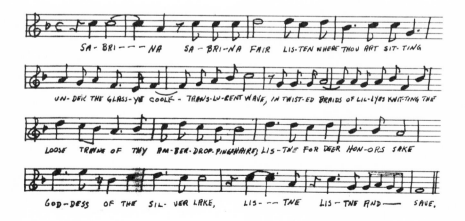

89

The verse [which follows] to singe or not.

Listen and appeare to us
In name of great *Oceanus,*
By th'earth shaking *Neptun's* mace
And *Tethys* grave majesticke pace,
 Eld. Bro. By hoarie *Nereus* wrincled looke,
And the *Carpathian* wisards hooke,
 2 Bro. By scalie *Tritons* winding shell,
And old sooth saying *Glaucus* spell,
 Eld. Bro. By *Leucothea's* lovely hands,
890 And her son that rules the strands,
 2 Bro. By *Thetis* tinsel-slipper'd feet,
And the songs of *Sirens* sweet,
 Eld. Bro. By dead *Parthenope's* deare tomb,
And faire *Ligea's* golden comb,
Wherewith she sits on diamond rocks
Sleeking her soft alluring locks,
 Dae. By all the *Nymphs* that nightly dance
Upon thy streams with wilie glance,
Rise, rise and heave thy rosie head
900 From thy coral-paven bed,
And bridle in thy headlong wave
Till thou our summons answerd have.
     Listen and save.   *[repeating the last*
                 phrase of the
                previous song.]

  Sabrina rises attended by water Nimphes and sings.

By the rushie fringed banke,
 Where growes the willow and the osier dancke
  My sliding chariot stayes,
 Thicke set with agat, and the azurne sheene
Of turkkis blew, and Emrould greene
 That in the channell strayes,
910 *Whilst from off the waters fleet*
 Thus I set my printlesse feet
 Ore the cowslips velvet head,
  That bends not as I tread,
 Gentle swaine at thy request
  I am here.

    Dae. Goddesse deare   *[Singing continues.]*
Wee implore thy powerfull hand
To undoe the charmed band
Of true virgin here distrest,
920   Through the force, and through the wile
Of unblest inchanter vile.
    Sab. Shepheard tis my office best
To helpe insnared chastitie;
Brightest Ladie looke on me,
Thus I sprinckle on thy brest   *[Sprinkles water.]*
Drops that from my fountaine pure
I have kept of precious cure.
Thrice upon thy fingers tip,   *[Again]*
Thrice upon thy rubied lip,
930   Next this marble venom'd seate
Smear'd with gummes of glutenous heate
I touch with chast palmes moist and cold,   *[Touches the chair]*
Now the spell hath lost his hold.
And I must hast ere morning houre
To waite in *Amphitrite's* bowre.

          Sabrina descends and the Ladie rises out
                    of her seate.

    Dae. Virgin, daughter of *Locrine*   *[Singing continues.]*
Sprung of old *Anchises* line
May thy brimmed waves for this
Their full tribute never misse
940   From a thousand pettie rills,
That tumble downe the snowie hills:
Summer drought, or singed aire
Never scorch thy tresses faire,
Nor wet Octobers torrent flood
Thy molten crystall fill with mudde,
May thy billowes rowle a shoare
The beryll, and the golden ore,
May thy loftie head be crown'd
With many a tower, and terrasse round,
950   And here and there thy banks upon
With groves of myrrhe, and cinnamon.

                            songe ends.

Come Ladie while heaven lends us grace,

91

Let us fly this cursed place,
Lest the sorcerer us intice
With some other new device.
Not a wast, or needlesse sound
Till we come to holyer ground,
I shall be your faithfull guide
Through this gloomie covert wide,
960 And not many furlongs thence
Is your Fathers residence,
Where this night are met in state
Many a freind to gratulate
His wish't presence, and beside
All the Swains that there abide,
With Jiggs, and rurall dance resort,
Wee shall catch them at their sport,
And our suddaine comming there
Will double all their mirth, and chere;
970 Come let us hast, the starrs are high
But night sits monarch yet in the mid skie.   *[Exeunt.]*

The sceane changes[;] then
is presented Ludlow towne
and the Presidents Castle,
then come in Countrie
daunces, and the like &c,
towards the end of those
sports the demon with the 2
brothers and the ladye come
in, the spiritt singes.

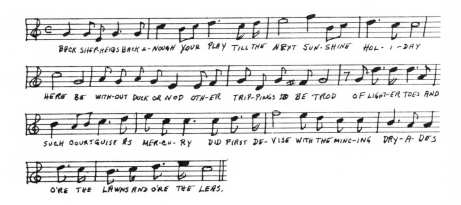

BACK SHEP-HERDS BACK A-NOUGH YOUR PLAY TILL THE NEXT SUN-SHINE HOL-I-DAY

HERE BE WITH-OUT DUCK OR NOD OTH-ER TRIP-PINGS TO BE TROD OF LIGHT-ER TOES AND

SUCH COURTGUISE AS MER-CU-RY DID FIRST DE-VISE WITH THE MINC-ING DRY-A-DES

O'RE THE LAWNS AND O'RE THE LEAS,

[The Daemon leads the children to where their parents
are seated in the audience
and in] This second song
praesents them to their
father and mother

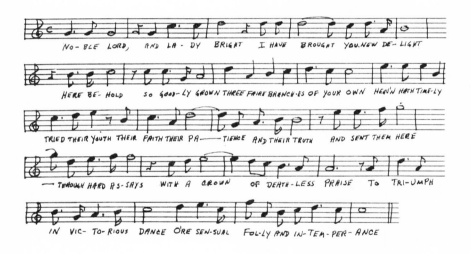

NO-BLE LORD, AND LA-DY BRIGHT I HAVE BROUGHT YOU NEW DE-LIGHT

HERE BE-HOLD SO GOOD-LY GROWN THREE FAIRE BRANCH-ES OF YOUR OWN HEAV'N HATH TIME-LY

TRIED THEIR YOUTH THEIR FAITH THEIR PA——TIENCE AND THEIR TRUTH AND SENT THEM HERE

—THROUGH HARD AS-SAYS WITH A CROWN OF DEATH-LESS PRAISE TO TRI-UMPH

IN VIC-TO-RIOUS DANCE O'RE SEN-SUAL FOL-LY AND IN-TEM-PER-ANCE

93

They dance [and everyone participates in the entertainments of the evening. At their conclusion,] the dances all ended[,] the Daemon [reenters in his sky robes and] singes or sayes

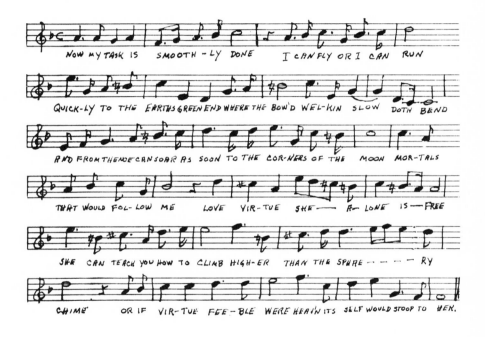

NOW MY TASK IS SMOOTH-LY DONE   I CAN FLY OR I CAN RUN

QUICK-LY TO THE EARTHS GREEN END WHERE THE BOW'D WEL-KIN SLOW DOTH BEND

AND FROM THENCE CAN SOAR AS SOON TO THE COR-NERS OF THE   MOON MOR-TALS

THAT WOULD FOL-LOW ME   LOVE   VIR-TUE   SHE —— A-LONE IS—FREE

SHE   CAN TEACH YOU HOW TO CLIMB HIGH-ER   THAN THE SPHRE — — — — RY

CHIME'   OR IF   VIR-TUE   FEE-BLE   WERE HEAV'N ITS SELF WOULD STOOP TO HER.

[Exit]

94

APPENDIX:
THE DATE AND OCCASION FOR
A MIDSUMMER NIGHT'S DREAM

Apart from a few unromantic dissidents, critics have seen *A Midsummer Night's Dream* as originally written to celebrate a wedding. The difficulty has been to identify which one, inasmuch as several in the 1590's can qualify, the two now most generally favored being those of Elizabeth Vere to William, Earl of Derby, on January 26, 1595; and of Elizabeth Carey to Thomas Berkeley on February 19, 1596.[1] Details in the play can fit either; and though Alexander and Brooks favor the later wedding for a variety of reasons—style and references to contemporary events—none proves to be a completely convincing resolution of the question.

The first two speeches of Theseus and Hippolyta which open the play, however, provide conclusive evidence not previously noticed in lines that have resisted a completely satisfactory explanation. The King of Athens is impatient for the arrival of his wedding day:

> Now, fair Hippolyta, our nuptial hour
> Draws on apace; four happy days bring in
> Another moon: but O, methinks, how slow
> This old moon wanes!   (I, i, 1-4)

She responds,

> Four days will quickly steep themselves in night;
> Four nights will quickly dream away the time;
> And then the moon, like to a silver bow
> New bent in heaven, shall behold the night
> Of our solemnities.   (7-11)

That is, in four days there will be a new moon. The marriage will take place on the fifth day. But why mention the *new* moon? Why the specificity of four and five days? Critics have generally ignored the former question and, for the latter, have assumed that Shakespeare, writing rapidly, may have vaguely imagined a play whose plot would take more time but actually wrote one which occupies only two days and did not bother to go back to rectify this minor mistake. As Brooks annotates, "The longer interval is wanted at this point to justify Theseus' impatience. The discrepancy, which does not trouble an audience and so did not trouble Shakespeare, is a minor instance of his 'double time'."

But let us assume that Theseus and Hippolyta represent in some sense the couple about to be married and in whose honor the play is being staged. In that case, Theseus is telling us that the performance of *Dream* takes place four days before the new moon; Hippolyta adds that the wedding itself will be the following day. We should follow Bottom's advice in the third act: "A calendar, a calendar! Look in the almanac; find out moonshine, find out moonshine!" Turning to the month of January, 1595, in G. Frende's *Almanack,* we discover that the new moon then was on the 30th, too late for the wedding of Elizabeth Vere and William Derby on the 26th. For those who prefer to think that the play celebrated the marriage of the Countess of Southampton to Sir Thomas Heneage on May 2, 1594, the new moon also came too late that month by over a week. But then moving on to 1596, in the month of February the new moon occurred on the 18th, the day before the wedding of Elizabeth Carey to Thomas Berkeley on the 19th, a perfect fit of dates.[2] That being the case, according to the testimony of the opening lines, *Dream* was first performed four days before the 18th—that is, on February 14, 1596, Saint Valentine's Day. One must remark on the complete suitability of its subject to the day as well as to the occasion.

This identification of Theseus with Thomas and Hippolyta with Elizabeth in the audience suggests a social background for his yet-unexplained statement,

> Hippolyta, I woo'd thee with my sword,
> And won thy love doing thee injuries;

96

> But I will wed thee in another key,
> With pomp, with triumph, and with revelling.   (I, i, 16-19)

This seems at best to be a tasteless comment and has been explained only by reference to its analogy in Chaucer's *Knight's Tale*. I should suggest instead that Theseus is recalling some social event in which Thomas and Elizabeth participated, probably lost now beyond recall, in which he "won" her. A mask or tournament modeled on the *Knight's Tale* seems most probable. Since John Smyth reports that the couple had developed affection for one another only since the previous autumn,[3] such an occasion would have taken place about then; Shakespeare must have known about it.

After the first nineteen lines of this first scene, however, the author makes no effort to accommodate the lunar date with the moonlight which floods the rest of the play, a fact that has perplexed many commentators. Quince, for instance, reports that the moon "doth shine that night" for their projected performance, whereas on February 14 it would have been in its latest phase. According to III, ii, 61 and 380, Venus is the morning star, whereas in the winter of 1596 it was actually visible only in the evening.[4] There are other discrepancies. The bad weather narrated by Titania in II, i, 88 ff. was actually the case in 1594 but not in 1596. Accordingly, years ago Chambers and Dover Wilson suggested that the first nineteen lines were written after the main part of the play and were inconsistently prefixed to it—as we can now say, for the February 14, 1596 performance.[5]

Of a similar problematic nature are allusions to May Day in IV, i, 102-103 and 130-131, which some have seen as a major support for the Southampton-Heneage wedding on May 2, 1594. As apt is Theseus's comment in the same scene that "Saint Valentine is past" (IV, i, 138), as indeed it is in the plot of the play staged the night of February 14, 1596. Furthermore, the hunting scene in which these allusions occur also connects directly with the groom's family. In its overview of the Berkeleys the main point which the *Dictionary of National Biography* makes about Thomas's father, Lord Henry, is that he was "a mighty hunter," the sport occupying him so completely as to have led to a (temporary) estrangement with the Queen a generation earlier. It is possible that Thomas, an only son, shared his

97

father's love of it which also so engrosses Theseus or that Shakespeare includes the father's interest in the characterization.

Some final consideration must be directed to the wedding ceremonies reported in the fourth act and their aftermath in the fifth. As has been seen, the play was staged on February 14, and the wedding itself celebrated five days later. But the exegencies of the plot required that the three couples be united so that the play of Pyramus and Thisbe could be presented to complete that plot. Accordingly, Quince reports that "the Duke is coming from the temple, and there is two or three lords and ladies more married" (IV, ii, 15-16). But *Dream* thereafter certainly does not exploit that event as, for instance, the last scene of *Merchant* does. For newly married couples the three groups of lovers make singularly little reference to the fact in Act 5. Theseus calls for the play of Pyramus and Thisbe not in its celebration but only

> To wear away this long age of three hours
> Between our after-supper and bed-time.   (V, i, 33-34)

Indeed, in this scene the only mention that a marriage has taken place is the question of the appropriateness of the choice of entertainment to "nuptials." The reason, of course, is that the actual performance of *Dream* took place five days before the wedding itself.

But at the end of the act there are three epilogues, one of which does explicitly concern the wedding. The performance on Valentine's Day would end with the Bergamask dance, followed by Theseus's eight-line epilogue—still with no mention that a marriage has been celebrated—and ending in its directive,

> A fortnight hold we this solemnity
> In nightly revels and new jollity.   (V, i, 355-356)

That is, the two weeks of festivities which are to climax on the 19th opened on Valentine's Day with the play (though they would close in only eleven days since in 1596 Ash Wednesday would come on February 25).

Then five days later at the end of the evening of the wedding, Puck made a possibly surprise appearance once more before

98

the guests to introduce Oberon and Titania again. Oberon had promised that they would

> *to-morrow* midnight, solemnly,
> Dance in Duke Theseus' house triumphantly,
> And bless it to all fair prosperity,   (IV, i, 87-89)

another inconsistency between the original play and Shakespeare's adaptation of it to the Carey-Berkeley nuptials. After the song and dance of the fairy masque Oberon and Titania bless the house and the newly married couple:

> To the best bride-bed [of Elizabeth and Thomas] will we,
> Which by us shall blessed be.   (V, i, 389-390)

The fairies then go on to prophecy,

> So shall all the couples three
> Ever true in loving be,   (393-394)

which in the context of the preceding play if spoken on February 14 would, of course, refer to Theseus-Hippolyta, Lysander-Hermia, and Demetrius-Helena. But if instead this epilogue was actually delivered late in the evening of February 19 after the wedding the three couples would be Sir George and Lady Elizabeth Carey, Lord Henry and Lady Katherine Berkeley, and the newly wed Thomas and Elizabeth. A few lines later it concludes with a prayer that the owner of the house, Sir George, "Ever shall in safety rest."[6] Shakespeare's company had been thriving under the patronage of Lord Hunsdon, Sir George's father, as they would under Sir George himself after his father's death later that year. Ten days before the performance of *Dream* their manager, James Burbage, had leased the property next door to the Carey home for a theatre (though it would be years before the public would be admitted; but a marriage performance of *Dream* could have taken place there). The fairy parts could well have been designed for the group of singing boys which Sir George maintained as part of his establishment; he would have directed arrangements for the evening, and Elizabeth was his only child.[7] Shakespeare could not have written the opening speeches of *Dream* until the wedding date had been set for February 19 and the performance for the 14th. It is by no means clear whether he adapted a text already under way or had conceived of the play all along as especially designed for the Carey-Berkeley celebration and made a few necessary late changes in some of its details to correspond with the date that the families finally settled on. In any case, the bride's father must have been well pleased—so well pleased that a year later he commissioned Shakespeare to write a play for another occasion, *The Merry Wives.*

NOTES

[1] See, for instance, E. K. Chambers, *William Shakespeare: A Study of Facts and Problems* (1930), I, 359, and his *Shakespearean Gleanings* (1946), p. 67; Peter Alexander, *Shakespeare's Life and Art* (1939), p. 105; and *A Midsummer Night's Dream,* ed. Harold F. Brooks (The New Arden Shakespeare, 1979), pp. lvi f. I follow the text of this edition. Elizabeth Carey was the niece of the recently widowed Dowager Countess of Derby, Alice Spencer.

[2] Several almanacs are readily available in the University Microfilm of the Short Title Catalogue, but I have not been able to locate either a copy or a microfilm of an almanac for 1596 and have extrapolated the date by proceeding from the last new moon of 1595. According to Frende it was on December 20. It would appear one day earlier for each of the succeeding two months, on January 19 and February 18. Anyone wishing to verify the various dates for the new moon should consult Herman H. Goldstein, *New and Full Moons, 1001 B.C. to A.D. 1651,* American Philosophical Society, 94 (1973).

[3] John Smyth, *The Berkeley Manuscripts: The Lives of the Berkeleys* (1883), II, 383, 395 ff. This collection is the authority for Lord Henry's passion for hunting to be considered below. Information about Thomas and his wedding is tantalizingly vague because he died before his father, Lord Henry, and so did not succeed to the title. Because of obvious references to her in *Dream* one would like to believe that Queen Elizabeth was present. As godmother to both Thomas and Elizabeth (as Smyth's manu-

scripts report), she would be likely to attend, but the fact seems to be beyond proof.

[4] Calculated from Bryant Tuckerman, *Planetary, Lunar, and Solar Positions A.D. 2 to A.D. 1649,* American Philosophical Society 59 (1964).

[5] See, e.g., Wilson's notes in the New Cambridge Edition (1924), p. 104.

[6] Puck's final speech in our present text was, of course, yet a third epilogue written to conclude the play as it was adapted to the public theatre, those for Valentine's Day and for the marriage day being omitted then.

[7] The facts are conveniently summarized from Chamber's original discoveries by Brooks, p. lvii.